Mastering Homeopathy 2

The Treatment of Irritable Bowel Syndrome

Title by the same author:

Mastering Homeopathy: Accurate Daily Prescribing for a Successful Practice (2004)

Mastering Homeopathy 2

The Treatment of Irritable Bowel Syndrome

Jon Gamble
BA, ND, Adv Dip Hom

Karuna Publishing

2006

First published in Australia by:
Karuna Publishing
122 Church Street
Wollongong, NSW, 2500
karuna@bigpond.net.au

Gamble, Jon.

Mastering homeopathy 2 : the treatment of irritable bowel syndrome.

1st ed.
Bibliography.
Includes index.
ISBN 0 9752473 1 0.

1. Homeopathy - Handbooks, manuals, etc. 2. Irritable colon - Treatment - Handbooks, manuals, etc. I. Title. (Series : Mastering homeopathy).

615.532

Printed in Australia by Griffin Press
Cover design by Tina Mulholland

Foreword

Jon's is a book founded on pathological prescribing and as such may seem to be opposed to principles like that of the single remedy and the totality of symptoms cherished by many homeopaths. My thought on this is that the spirit of the law gives life and the letter of the law kills. Principles that are adhered to the exclusion of consistent results require us to re-examine our attitude and understanding.

Jon elucidates many cases where he has used a single medicine or a series of medicines and sometimes alternating medicines, to solve cases of IBS. He also relates the use of these various medicines to specific causal factors of each individual's symptoms. In this way he is carrying on the tradition of intelligent pathological prescribing introduced to this country largely by Alan Jones and Dr. Parimal Banerji. The successful use of this system makes it evident that remedies have a specific physiological action which, while integrated with mental and general symptoms, may be considered independently in regard to their action on specific diseases in many cases.

In Chapter 3 Jon states "pathology must be treated before a 'mentals' prescription" and gives a case with fear and night terrors with IBS which Stramonium won't cure. I agree with the spirit of this principle excepting where the medicine is capable of curing both the mental and the physical symptoms through its known action, or its understood action, via the modern systems such as those recommended by Drs. Sankaran and Scholten.

There are many ways into a case and in my opinion many medicines that can assist in a certain disease. They include finding the mental or feeling association with the pathology such as Sankaran's method of vital sensation, Boenninghausen's methodology and defined pathological prescribing. Jon's work is centred on the latter but uses as an adjunct constitutional prescribing with standard known medicines like Silica, Lycopodium and Phosphorus. His approach to treating 'the exogenous disease phenomena' before the 'constitution' appears to be correct in IBS, just as it has been proven correct in many other treatments that are 'Never well since' a specific infection.

Jon has elucidated the many categories of IBS: Intestinal parasitosis; candida albicans; emotional; food sensitivity; post viral etc. and the cure of each category with homeopathic medicines. Such a thorough clinical study of a common disease together with effective treatment protocols such as he presents challenges modern medicine to such a degree that in time, with further clinical verification, it should replace it as the proper treatment for IBS.

He has also proposed that parasitosis is one of the 'invisible morbific influences' which Hahnemann first described and as such should be a new miasm requiring specific medicines. There is ample evidence for this considering the prevalence of this disease syndrome and its illustrated clinical practicality. How this relates to other modern miasmatic theories is a mystery that will only be resolved with time.

Jon has produced an admirable foundation work for the treatment of Irritable Bowel Syndrome. It is a boon for all homeopaths in that it makes the protocol more clearly understandable and more easily defined in homeopathic terms. Such clear clinical methodology is of outstanding practical benefit to our profession and the confidence to practitioners and patients alike.

Peter Tumminello

Contents

Foreword...5
Preface...9
Introduction...11

Chapter 1: Irritable Bowel Syndrome: Diagnostic Criteria and Causes...15

Chapter 2: Differential Diagnosis...39

Chapter 3: The Treatment of Irritable Bowel Syndrome...49
- Category 1: Intestinal Parasitosis...51
- Category 2: Dysbiosis & Candida of the GIT...61
- Category 3: Emotional...63
- Category 4: Food Sensitivity...67
- Category 5: 'Never Well Since'...69
- Category 6: Hypochlorhydria & Gastro-Oesophageal Reflux..71
- Category 7: Gallbladder Stasis...74
- Category 8: Gastritis & Peptic Ulcer...75
- Category 9: Post Viral...77
- Category 10: Constipation...79
- Category 11: Diarrhoea & Faecal Incontinence...80
- Category 12: Diet & Lifestyle...82
- Category 13: Bowel Nosodes...83
- Category 14: Particular symptoms: no other cause found...86
- Category 15: Cellular Memory...87

Chapter 4: Cases...91

Chapter 5: Choosing the Order of Treatment...136

Chapter 6: A Parasitic Miasm...141

Chapter 7: Frequently Asked Questions...147

Appendices
1: Rome Criteria...150
2: Intestinal Parasites...151

Bibliography...152

Index of Medicines...154

General Index...155

Acknowledgements...158

Preface

Many practitioners using my previous book, *Accurate Daily Prescribing for a Successful Practice*, suggested that I focus on a specific topic in greater detail. The present book is a result of that suggestion.

In this work I introduce a controversial proposition. It is this: 70 per cent of people with Irritable Bowel Syndrome can be significantly treated with only five different homeopathic medicines. People in this group all have the same miasmatic cause of their illness. It is one of the invisible, morbific and contagious agents, which Hahnemann was not able to fully identify at the time of his writing. Had he lived in the age of microbiology, then his classification of the miasms may have been quite different.

While this proposition may be controversial, it is based on clinical experience, not philosophy. It is also supported by medical research completed independent of my own clinic.

J.C.G.
August 2006

For Beryl and Jeff

Introduction

Irritable Bowel Syndrome is a modern enigma. Since the causes of IBS are largely unknown, its treatment is filled with guesswork, with diagnostic tests used less often than is needed. Treatment revolves around managing symptoms with antispasmodics or bulking agents.

Consequently, IBS continues to be an ever increasing presentation in clinic, with many patients showing frustration with their failure to recover. It is therefore a homeopath's challenge to provide good clinical outcomes.

What is IBS?
While theories abound as to aetiology and management, modern medicine seems to be more focused on what the patient's symptoms are *not*. It is of course important to rule out more serious pathologies with medical investigations. If none of these are positive, IBS is the likely diagnosis. IBS thus lies at the bottom of the diagnostic barrel, yet it is meaningless as such a diagnosis offers few clues to the most appropriate treatment for the patient.

In complementary medicine, a large emphasis is placed on gut dysbiosis, the imbalance of gut flora allowing proliferation of pathogenic organisms. Consequently there are a number of over-the-counter products for IBS. Some contain lactobacilli, which may help to counter gut dysbiosis. Others contain herbs such as peppermint oil, intended to reduce flatulence and colic. These self-help measures inevitably involve guess work, especially if the patient has not been correctly diagnosed. One test which is not performed enough in IBS is a diagnostic stool sample. A stool assessment can show the presence of many pathogens which are a major cause of IBS. This is discussed in depth in Chapters 1 and 3.

What causes IBS?
IBS is caused by no single entity. It is a cluster of symptoms with multiple causes all placed under the generic term of IBS. Some of these causes are more common than others, which explains the difficulty in successfully managing IBS. When IBS has multiple causes, it is difficult for one medicine, whether prescribed or

over-the-counter, to fully address those causes. If there is a single cause of the IBS, as some of the cases in this book demonstrate, there still needs to be a clear assessment of the cause before an effective medicine can be used.

For clarity, I have given each of these causes a category and referred to each of them in that way, for example, 'Category 3 IBS'. Some patients' IBS may consist of more than one disease category at once. Of the 15 categories I have listed, most are clear causes of the IBS, while some are descriptors of treatment approaches from a homeopathic perspective.

Materia Medica for IBS

The medicines and potencies in this book essentially constitute a particular *Materia Medica* for the treatment of IBS. Most of these medicines are well known by homeopaths. What is not well known are some of their specific uses in treating IBS. For example, *Cina* is known is a medicine for irritable children. In this work I also present it as a major treatment for adult IBS. *Cina* also treats anxiety and insomnia in adults, when associated with IBS.

How often would we think that anxiety and insomnia arise from a gut problem? As homeopaths we often have a strong focus on the mental symptoms. As I have found in my practice, this can lead us to miss physical causes of emotional disturbance.

Since I am presenting a very specific *Materia Medica*, largely based on clinical experience, I have not used any of the traditional Repertories in preparing this work. That is because many of the aspects of the medicines I discuss are under-represented in the Repertories. To use the above example, the *Repertory* only grades *Cina* with a '1' under Mind, Anxiety. As you will see, it has a far wider scope when there is anxiety with gut disturbance. I have found it more effective in practice to approach IBS treatment from the perspective of causative categories, and treatment protocols that I have described.

Posology

Most of the treatment protocols in this book recommend repetition of the medicine in a specific potency every second day for at least one month. This gives consistent results. It was from Dr Parimal Banerji of Calcutta that I first learned specificity of potency and repetition of medicines in certain diseases and that thinking is reflected here.

However, when prescribing constitutionally I give far less of the medicine, and usually in a higher potency. This is in keeping with a more classical orientation and a perception of the level of sensitivity between the patient and the medicine they are to take.

All potency references in this book, eg *Nux vom 30,* refer to the centesimal scale, unless otherwise stated. References to the male gender, except in the case studies, are made for convenience but equally apply to the female gender.

Chapter 1
Irritable Bowel Syndrome: Diagnostic Criteria, Causes & Categories

Contents

What is Irritable Bowel Syndrome?...16
Lifestyle Factors…18
Diagnosis…19
On Examination…19
Causes & Categories…19
    Category 1: Intestinal Parasitosis…20
    Category 2: Dysbiosis & Candida of the GIT…23
    Category 3: Emotional…24
    Category 4: Food Sensitivity…25
    Category 5: 'Never Well Since'…27
    Category 6: Hypochlorhydria & Gastro-Oesophageal Reflux..28
    Category 7: Gallbladder Stasis…29
    Category 8: Gastritis & Peptic Ulcer…30
    Category 9: Post Viral…31
    Category 10: Constipation…32
    Category 11: Diarrhoea & Faecal Incontinence…34
    Category 12: Diet & Lifestyle…35
    Category 13: Bowel Nosodes…36
    Category 14: Particular symptoms: no other cause found…36
    Category 15: Cellular Memory…37

What is Irritable Bowel Syndrome?

Irritable Bowel Syndrome (IBS) refers to *shifting abdominal pain with alternating constipation and diarrhoea.* This is sometimes described as irregular or disturbed bowel function. One of these symptoms alone may be the prominent one which compels a patient to seek treatment. There may be pain with either constipation or diarrhoea, but more commonly, IBS refers to this alternation between constipation and diarrhoea, where the pain is shifting. While the pain is often confined to one quadrant of the abdomen, it is not always in precisely the same location. Pain relief from passing flatus is found only in some patients.

Diagnostic Features of IBS

IBS has recurrent abdominal pain plus two or more of:

- Pain better from defecation
- Altered stool at the onset of pain
- Abdominal bloating
- Increased or decreased stools at the onset of pain
- A 'never completely empty' sensation after passing stool
- Passing mucus from the rectum
- Morning cluster of motions
- Constipation alternating with diarrhoea[1]

---

[1] Compare the Manning Criteria:
Irritable bowel syndrome if ≥3 are present:

- Abdominal pain
- Relief of pain on defecation
- Increased stool frequency with pain
- Looser stools with pain
- Mucus in stools
- Feeling of incomplete evacuation

See also the Rome II criteria in Appendix 1

Other symptoms reported by patients with IBS:

- Fatigue (some IBS patients also have Chronic Fatigue Syndrome)
- Nausea
- Unexplained insomnia or disturbed sleep patterns
- Susceptibility to colds, flus, sinusitis or post-nasal drip
- Headaches
- Allergic sensitivity
- Restless leg syndrome
- Gastric reflux
- Crawling skin.

Patients are sometimes diagnosed with IBS even though they do not have the above specific symptoms. In practice, IBS has become a generic term for the presence of abdominal pain with variable bowel habits, once pathology tests have excluded other causes. Some of the 'red flag' symptoms in abdominal pain are listed below. With the rare exception of weight loss and fever (See Category 1 IBS), the symptoms below are not IBS and always require further evaluation:

- Weight loss
- Blood in stools
- Anaemia
- Fever.

If the patient is over 50 and presents with altered bowel function, medical evaluation is always recommended.

It is also helpful, at least from a treatment perspective, to classify IBS as either constipation- or diarrhoea-dominant, since this will greatly affect the treatment plan.

When patients present for homeopathic treatment, many have already had a normal colonoscopy to exclude pathology. IBS is therefore considered to be a *functional* disturbance rather than a pathology.

Lifestyle Factors in IBS

Lifestyle factors may include:

- Stress
- Excessive use of caffeine
- Inadequate water intake
- Inadequate sleep
- Long working hours without finding time for toileting
- Poor nutrition
- Lack of exercise
- Eating meals too quickly (thus swallowing air).

Stress

IBS is often stress related, but so are any other functional illnesses, such as migraines or period pain. While it is easy to dismiss IBS as just 'stress', in some cases emotional factors are clearly causative. A patient's symptoms may disappear on weekends or holidays. A stressful work environment may be the only identifiable cause of symptoms. Therefore, one might then conclude that the IBS is a stress related functional disturbance. One specialist IBS clinic claims that 51% of female IBS patients reported a past history of life threatening physical trauma.[2] In other cases antidepressants (eg *Amitriptyline*) improve IBS.

Diet

Eating large, infrequent meals can put significant pressure on the digestive system, and is a possible factor in indigestion and reflux. Similarly, under-eating, if severe, may lead to malnutrition, disturbance to metabolism and energy, and may be a result of, or lead to, psychological disorders. IBS is sometimes improved by correction of the diet. If lack of dietary fibre is considered to be a cause, the addition of dietary fibre should proceed for at least one week before re-assessment.

---

[2] Jacques Duff, Behavioural Neurotherapy Clinic, Melbourne: www.ibs-irritable-bowel-syndrome.com.au

Diagnosis

The following should be checked before a diagnosis of IBS is made:

- Food sensitivity testing
- Coeliac screening: Gliadin antibody test or IgA antibodies to transglutaminase[3]
- History, lifestyle, dietary factors
- If any 'red flag' symptoms (see above), make appropriate referrals.

For a full differential diagnosis see Chapter 2.

On examination

Palpation may reveal a tender (spastic) colon or a loaded colon if there is constipation. The patient may experience pain anywhere in the abdomen, including the upper right quadrant (hepatic flexure) or the upper left quadrant (splenic flexure) when there is constipation. While the pain is most often felt in the descending colon, it may be referred from any location in the abdomen.

Causes and Categories of IBS

I have found it useful to categorise 15 types of IBS, as detailed below. These categories may be diagnostic, for example intestinal parasites as in Category 1, or offer a particular treatment where no other seems relevant, as in Category 13 IBS. These categories are not exclusive: there is overlap found with most IBS cases, each of which may need a sequential treatment protocol.

[3] There is now an instant finger-prick test manufactured by Biotech: www.anibiotech.fi

Category 1: Intestinal Parasitosis

Evidence of Parasitic IBS

Our clinic audit shows 70 per cent of IBS cases display a sensitivity to, or have symptoms suggesting, intestinal parasites. Only a small number of these patients are able to date their symptoms from a previous episode of gastroenteritis or traveller's diarrhoea. One study suggests that infectious gastroenteritis is associated with an 11-fold increase in the risk of developing IBS.[4] The majority of cases, however, have no recorded (or remembered) acute episode of diarrhoea. Indeed, any colonisation of the bowel by pathogens has not necessarily had an acute onset. An asymptomatic patient with pre-existing gut dysbiosis will be predisposed to intestinal parasites because the disturbance to normal gut flora undermines the gut's functional immunity.

Dr Tom Borody, director of Centre for Digestive Diseases in Sydney, says many patients with IBS have the parasites dientamoeba fragilis or blastocystis hominis which, in Australia, are more common than giardia. According to Borody, laboratory detection requires a special fixative stool test which prevents degradation (as compared to fresh stool test which does not show the organism).[5] In one study, patients in the controlled clinical trial displayed these symptoms:

- Irregular bowel habits
- Bloating & cramping
- Diarrhoea or constipation
- Nausea, fatigue, anorexia.

Adults were given *Doxycycline* and *Iodoquinol*; and children were given *Flagyl* and *Iodoquinol* (or placebo). 67 per cent of patients receiving these drugs reported significant improvement in all symptoms.[6] This is in accord with my own clinical findings where we use a homeopathic anti-parasitic medicine for IBS treatment.

---

[4] *American Journal of Gastroenterology* 2003; 98:1970-75
[5] Reported in *Medical Observer*, 11.10.02
[6] Reported in *Medical Observer*, 11.10.02

Reliable testing for parasites

One problem with achieving an accurate diagnosis of intestinal parasites is reliable pathology testing. As stated by Borody, above, one specialist pathology laboratory in Melbourne[7] says that due to the lifecycle of parasites such as blastocystis hominis, the parasites may not be present in every stool. For this reason, testing over a 3-day period is necessary. Specialist laboratories recommend the use of a special fixative when collecting stool samples, without which the evidence of parasites may degrade before the sample reaches the laboratory.[8] Eosinophilia will be found in some cases of intestinal parasitosis and can therefore alert one to the need for a stool test.

Dysbiosis & parasitosis

We know that a low level of the normal beneficial bacteria (gut dysbiosis) can lead to the proliferation of opportunistic pathogens, both bacteria and fungi, which are normal gut residents. These are normally kept in check by the beneficial bacteria. Dysbiosis may also facilitate infestation by intestinal parasites (ie organisms foreign to the human gut). But it is not always known what came first: did gut dysbiosis create the environment for parasitic infestation or did the parasites enter the gut and digest the beneficial bacteria?

Some Common Intestinal Parasites

- Ancylostoma canium (dog hookworm loves to burrow through the skin of those who walk barefoot in tropical areas)
- Blastocystis hominis
- Cryptosporidium parnum
- Dientamoeba fragilis
- Entamoeba histolytica (can be misdiagnosed as Inflammatory Bowel Disease when it causes chronic amoebic colitis)
- Fasciolopsis buskii
- Giardia
- Strongyloides sterc
- Taenia
- Toxoplasmosis gondii
- Trichinella

---

[7] ARL Pathology, Melbourne, Australia www.arlaus.com.au

[8] ARL Pathology, Melbourne (above) and Histopath Specialist Pathologists in Sydney use a special fixative to preserve parasites at viable room temperature: histopath@tpg.com.au

Symptoms:

Adults or children will have one or more of the following symptoms:

- Abdominal pain especially umbilical
- Allergies (including colds and flus)
- Anaemia
- Anorexia
- Anxiety*
- Bloating
- Constipation*
- Diarrhoea*
- Emaciation
- Fatigue
- Flatulence
- Flushes of heat
- Insomnia
- Irritability*
- Nasal itch*
- Nausea
- Night terrors*
- Nocturnal fever*
- Rectal itch*
- Restless leg syndrome
- Skin itch or 'crawling'
- Teeth grinding*
- Variable appetite*
- Weakness
- Weight loss

*These symptoms are commonly found in children

Children & IBS

I have found that in almost every case, a child presenting with any of the above symptoms will have intestinal parasites. Frequently children with intestinal parasites will have irritability or nightmares. Children with ongoing diarrhoea, steatorrhoea and poor weight gain should of course be assessed for Coeliac Disease: see Chapter 2.

Constipation & Diarrhoea

While diarrhoea is an acknowledged symptom of intestinal parasitosis, it is less well known that constipation may also be generated, or worsened by, the presence of parasites. In any event, it is clear from a perusal of the above symptoms that parasites have an effect on the nervous system, which can result in mood disorders.

Category 2: Dysbiosis & Candida of the GIT

Candidiasis of the gut is commonly found in women who have a history of vaginal candida (monilia). It is not an intestinal parasite. Intestinal parasites are foreign organisms, not comprising the normal bowel flora of humans. Candida is a normal organism found in the human gut which has proliferated because of ongoing use of antibiotics, the contraceptive pill or other cause.

The use of antibiotics predisposes to candida overgrowth. Antibiotics destroy many of the beneficial bacteria in the gut, but do not affect candida albicans. Consequently, candida able to proliferate since it is not kept in check by normal gut flora.

Overgrowth of opportunistic *bacterial* pathogens also occurs in gut dysiosis. Overgrowth of proteus, streptococcus and staphylococcus are thought to contribute to IBS symptoms.[9]

Symptoms:

- Abdominal bloating & flatulence
- Sugar and carbohydrate craving and/or intolerance
- Mood swings
- History of thrush or vaginitis
- Fatigue.

---

[9] Campbell-McBride, N, *Gut and Psychology Syndrome,* Medinform Publishing, Cambridge, UK, 2004, p 31

Category 3: Emotional

As already elucidated by the medical profession, emotional stress plays a large part in aetiologies of IBS. One study concluded that 97 per cent of those in the study experienced worsening of their symptoms when exposed to emotional stressors. [10] Relaxation techniques or oral nervine aids may play a part in reducing symptom severity, however these do not offer a cure. Another study found that Cognitive Behavioural Therapy enhanced the treatment of IBS patients who were taking antispasmodic medication.[11]

Symptoms:

- *IBS symptoms +*
- *Symptoms are aggravated during times of stress*
- *Symptoms may be better during sleep*
- *Thinking about symptoms may worsen them.*

---

[10] Study at Royal North Shore Hospital, Sydney, reported in *Gut*, 1998; 43:256-61.

[11] Kennedy, T, et al, "Cognitive Behavioural Therapy in addition to antispasmodic treatment for irritable bowel syndrome in primary care: randomized clinical trial" *BMJ* 2005; 331:435

Category 4: Food Sensitivity

Patients may have undiagnosed lifelong food sensitivities, the most common of which are:

- Wheat and gluten
- Cow's milk products
- Yeast
- Salicylates.

Leaky gut & dysbiosis

Food sensitivity is thought to arise from 'leaky gut syndrome'. Leaky gut is an increase in the permeability of the intestinal mucosa to luminal macromolecules, antigens and toxins. This can be associated with inflammatory, degenerative and/or atrophic mucosal damage. Dysbiosis may be a predisposing factor to leaky gut, and can result from the use of:

- Antibiotics
- Antacids
- Analgaesics.

Stress

It is also postulated that prolonged emotional stress can predispose to both dysbiosis and leaky gut. Both may cause symptoms suggestive of food sensitivity.[12]

Food sensitivity can also be caused by the presence of intestinal parasites, even if there is no pre-disposing dysbiosis. When the parasites are removed the food sensitivity improves.

Gut inflammation->constipation & diarrhoea->stress cycle

The regular consumption of foods to which one is sensitive may cause chronic gut inflammation. Serotonin and acetylcholine, which play a significant part in gastrointestinal motility, may be affected by the chronic inflammation. This may lead to either constipation or diarrhoea, which could therefore be seen as a neurological problem. If it were not so, then emotional stress could play no part in the manifestation of these symptoms. Anyone who has experienced

---

[12] See generally Campell-McBride, N, *Gut and Psychology Syndrome,* Medinform Publishing, Camridge, UK, 2004

diarrhoea before public speaking knows that there is a clear relationship! It is possible for gastrointestinal disorders to both cause, and be caused by, emotional stress. Consequent chronic mood disorders are also a possible result of gastrointestinal dysfunction. Our vernacular represents this understanding when we use expressions such as 'I have a gut feeling that.....'.

Other common causes of what appears to be food sensitivity symptoms are gallbladder stasis and hypochlorhydria.

Symptoms:

- In addition to other symptoms, there is aggravation of symptoms following a certain food or food group
- In leaky gut, symptoms may also be emotional and behavioural (eg, think of how child behaviour is influenced by food colourings).

Category 5: 'Never Well Since'

The onset of the IBS may date from a specific previous illness event, such as surgery, allopathic medication, or another event, for example:

- Abdominal surgery
- Antibiotic use
- Glandular fever (Infectious Mononucleosis)
- Oral Contraceptive Pill (OCP)
- Other bacterial or viral diseases

Symptoms:

- There are no symptoms specific to this category. Diagnosis is made solely from the patient's history, noting a cascade of symptoms since a specific event.

Category 6 : Hypochlorhydria & Gastro-oesophageal Reflux

A significant proportion of IBS patients also experience gastric reflux as part of their symptom picture. Reflux may be caused by hypochlorhydria (insufficient stomach acid).

Symptoms:

- IBS symptoms as described +
- Heartburn (sharp or burning pain) felt at the cardiac orifice, oesophagus, trachea or larynx
- Dysphagia
- Voice loss or croaky voice
- Regurgitation and/or excessive burping
- Sensation of tightness around the throat
- Abdominal bloating
- Belching and full sensation after eating if there is hypochlorhydria.

Category 7: Gallbladder Stasis

Sludge of the bile duct is a not uncommon cause of the symptoms below, as is gallbladder calculi. Unlike calculi, sludge is not evident on ultrasound, and can be best diagnosed on the presenting symptoms. Gallbladder stasis is usually a concomitant factor, not a sole cause, of IBS.

Symptoms:

- Pale stools
- Nausea
- Afternoon headaches
- Fatty food intolerance
- Dull epigastric pain
- Dull pain in right hypochondrium.

Category 8: Gastritis & Peptic Ulcer

Some IBS patients also experience gastric symptoms as part of their IBS symptom picture. If reflux and/or hypochlorhydria are chronic, gastritis and ulceration can result. While the symptoms are similar to Category 6, with gastritis and ulcer the disease has progressed into a pathology.

Symptoms:

- IBS symptoms as described +:
- Heartburn (sharp or burning pain) felt at cardiac orifice, epigastrium, oesophagus, trachea or larynx
- Dysphagia
- Voice loss or croaky voice
- Cough and/or mucus in the larynx, sometimes rising to the posterior nares
- Regurgitation and/or excessive burping with or without pain
- Sensation of tightness or lump in the throat
- Bloating.

Category 9: Post Viral

There is a small group of cases whose IBS symptoms appear to be post-viral.

This category is a significant cause of IBS which does not appear to have been recognised in allopathic medicine.

Patients in this category demonstrate IBS symptoms which have an acute, cyclical onset. Their symptoms may appear, for example, once per month, and last for many days to one or two weeks. They are largely free of bowel symptoms between attacks, yet they complain of generally feeling unwell, having excessive fatigue, or vague nausea. The acute attacks often consist of severe abdominal cramps and diarrhoea. These cases can easily be confused with intestinal parasitosis. Antiparasitic medicines given to these patients will afford no relief, and may worsen the case.

Symptoms:

- IBS symptoms as described +:
- Fatigue
- Nausea
- Repeated colds, flus or throat infections (a sign of lowered immunity)
- Clear onset of symptoms with or soon after a viral infection.
- Ongoing cyclic diarrhoea or abdominal cramps
- Migraine
- Unexplained myalgia.

Category 10: Constipation

Misuse of laxatives and lack of dietary bulk (fibre) may cause a 'lazy' bowel, with inadequate peristalsis and muscle spasm. Constipation may also be a result of intestinal parasitosis and gut dysbiosis. I suspect that emotional stress is a factor more often than is commonly recognised. Many patients with constipation relate how they have a history of 'holding on' until they arrived home to go to the toilet.

Symptoms:

- Less than one bowel motion per day
- Overflow symptoms, with small amounts of stool being passed, which may be loose
- No urge for stool
- Ineffectual urging for stool.

Causes of Constipation
Not all constipation is IBS related, particularly if caused by one of the factors below.

Lifestyle

- Inadequate fluid intake
- Insufficient exercise
- Problems relating to toileting, ie too busy to go to the toilet particularly first thing in the morning
- Poor diet, lacking in fruit, vegetables and fibre.

Central Nervous System Disorders

- CVA
- Brain tumours
- Parkinson's disease
- Depression
- Dementia
- Multiple sclerosis
- Spinal cord lesions
- Cauda equine lesions
- Shy-Drager Syndrome

Allopathic Drugs

- Analgesics particularly those containing codeine
- Opiates
- Antacids
- Antispasmodics
- Antidepressants
- Antipsychotics
- Anti-parkinsonian medications
- Anti-diarrhoeal agents
- Anticonvulsants
- Anti-inflammatory agents
- Mineral overdoses

Metabolic or Endocrine Disturbances

- Hypothyroidism
- Diabetes
- Hypercalcaemia
- Hypokalaemia
- Porphyria

Miscellaneous

- Pregnancy
- Immobility (bed rest etc)[13].

[13] Ratnaike, Ranjit, "How to Treat: Constipation", *Australian Doctor,* 17.9.99, I-VIII

Category 11: Diarrhoea & Faecal Incontinence

Inappropriate diet or food sensitivity may predispose to diarrhoea. Too much dietary fibre in some constitutions may be one reason. Diarrhoea from dietary fibre can indicate gut dysbiosis. Diarrhoea is often caused by intestinal parasites, as already described.

Non-IBS Diarrhoea
Causes of faecal incontinence and diarrhoea which are not related to IBS are:

- Congenital
- Obstetric
- Constipation overflow (faecal impaction appears as diarrhoea)
- Neurological disease
- Rectal prolapse
- Iatrogenic trauma to anal sphincter
- Post-colon and rectal surgery
- Spinal trauma
- Idiopathic.[14]

Symptoms:

- Unformed or partially formed, urgent stool.

[14] Rieger, Nicholas, "How to Treat: Faecal Incontinence", *Australian Doctor,* 6.9.02, I-VII

Category 12: Diet & Lifestyle

Some 'IBS' can be corrected simply with dietary and lifestyle adjustments. Skipping meals and reliance on convenience foods will result in inadequate nutrition and disturbance to bowel habits. Taking vitamins may assist with nutritional deficiencies, but regular meals which include fresh fruit and vegetables plus plenty of fluids are essential for normal bowel function.

Therefore, inappropriate lifestyle habits must also be considered, for example, the use of regular recreational drugs. An inappropriate working environment may lead to disease. For example, a person prone to insomnia should not work night shifts, but requires a regulated sleeping routine.

Lifestyle factors may include:

- Excessive use of caffeine
- Inadequate water intake
- Inadequate sleep
- Long working hours
- Poor nutrition
- Lack of exercise
- Eating meals too quickly (thus swallowing air)
- Not following one's urge to go to the toilet – ie too busy.

The eating of large infrequent meals may put significant pressure on the digestive system, and is a possible factor in indigestion and reflux. Similarly, under-eating, if severe, may lead to malnutrition, disturbed metabolism and energy, and may be a result of, or lead to, psychological disorders.

Category 13: Bowel Nosodes

Category 14: Particular Symptoms: no other cause found

The above two categories are not causes of IBS. They represent particular treatment methods where the cause of IBS cannot be identified.

Category 15: Cellular Memory

My current thinking is that where a patient has been treated for intestinal parasites yet their symptoms persist in the same or altered form, this may to be the cellular memory of the chronic disease which leaves a residual affect in the nervous system.

The nerves in the bowel wall are so used to responding to the chronic inflammation or parasitic infection that they are reacting *as though the parasitic infection is still present.*

Chapter 2
Differential Diagnosis

This summary is confined to presentations of mid to lower abdominal pain as differential diagnoses to IBS.

Contents

Addison's disease...40
Aerophagy...40
Appendicitis...40
Candida Albicans (& gut dysbiosis)...40
Carcinoid Syndrome...41
Coeliac Disease...41
Colonic Carcinoma...42
Crohn's Disease...43
Diverticulitis...43
Embolic Injury to Bowel...43
Gynaecological...44
Haemorrhagic Colitis...45
Hernia...45
Inflammatory Bowel Disease...45
Ischaemic Colitis...46
Pancreatic Carcinoma...46
Peritonitis...46
Rectal Mucosal Prolapse...46
Sub-acute Bowel Obstruction...46
Thyrotoxicosis...47
Ulcerative Colitis...47
Zollinger-Ellison Syndrome...48

Shortlist of Symptom Differentials...48

Addison's disease

Symptoms:
- Diarrhoea
- Generalised skin pigmentation including surgical scars, buccal tissue and skin creases
- Hypotension and weakness.

Assessment
Blood chemistry and haematology.

Aerophagy

Symptoms:
- Distention of the abdomen with frequent belching associated with oesophageal reflux.

Appendicitis

Symptoms:
- Right (sometimes left) abdominal pain
- Vomiting after the pain is established
- Fever
- Nausea
- Headache.

Assessment
Positive rebound test and local pain.

Candida albicans (Monilia) colonisation of the GIT

GIT candidiasis is commonly found in women who suffer from vaginal candida (monilia). GIT candida symptoms can be similar to hypoglycaemic symptoms. Where the patient has tiredness and dizziness or headache more than two hours after eating with a craving for sugar, one should think of a disturbance in sugar metabolism rather than candidiasis. If there is a history of vaginal candidiasis with leucorrhoea or itching, then think of GIT candida. Of course, both syndromes may occur concurrently. Treatment of candida is discussed elsewhere.[15]

Symptoms:

- Abdominal bloating and flatulence
- Sugar craving and/or intolerance
- Mood swings
- History of thrush or vaginitis
- Fatigue.

Assessment

A finger prick test which can be performed in any clinic is now available. Local swab culture in the event of oral or genital candida.

Carcinoid syndrome

Symptoms:

- Diarrhoea

Findings:

- Liver secondaries

Coeliac Disease

Coeliac Disease refers to a patient with gluten allergy.

Symptoms:

- Malabsorption causing foul smelling stool and weight loss (or weight gain in some cases)
- Bloating
- Reflux
- Pallor
- Diarrhoea or constipation
- Anaemia
- Steatorrhoea
- Thyroid disease
- Migraine

[15] Gamble, J, *Mastering Homeopathy: Accurate Daily Prescribing for a Successful Practice,* Karuna Publishing, Wollongong, Australia, 2004

- Osteoporosis, osteopaenia or unexplained bone fracture (due to malabsorption of minerals)[16]
- Increased risk of gastrointestinal malignancy (where gluten is not properly screened from diet)
- Dental enamel defects
- Joint pain
- Fatigue, weakness or lack of energy
- Depression
- Aphthous ulcers
- Skin lesions (eg dermatitis herpetiformis has blistering, itchy skin with symmetrical distribution on the face, elbows, knees and buttock).

Assessment:
The Gliadin Antibody Assay will indicate positive gliadin antibodies in Coeliac Disease. Other assessments: Tissue Transglutaminase Antibody Assay (tTG) test; biopsy via colonoscopy. A finger-prick test is now available.

Colonic carcinoma

Symptoms:

- Abdominal mass may be palpable
- Pallor
- Weight loss
- Intermittent rectal bleeding.

Assessments:
CT scan and colonoscopy. Look for liver secondaries and iron deficiency anaemia.

[16] Rouse, R, "Suspect Coeliac after Non-Axial Fracture", *Medical Observer,* 15.10.04

Crohn's Disease (Regional Ileitis)

Symptoms:

- Right iliac fossa or central colicky pain with localised tenderness
- Weight loss
- Abdominal mass may be present
- Perianal fissures or fistula
- Swollen skin tags.

Findings:
Local peritoneal irritation, perforation, haemorrhage and structuring, often confined to the terminal ileum.

Assessments:
Blood study, barium meal x-ray, colonoscopy.

Diverticulitis

Symptoms:

- Increasing pain in left iliac fossa
- Fever
- Anorexia
- Constipation or diarrhoea.

Embolic injury to the bowel

Ischaemia of the bowel caused by embolus.

Symptoms:

- Vague mid-abdominal ache with increasing peritonism, acidosis then shock.

Compare: Ischaemic colitis.

Gynaecological:

1. Mittelschmerz

Symptoms:
- Acute, mid-cycle, severe pain in left or right iliac fossa which rapidly abates after 6-24 hours, which can occur monthly.
- Mild fever.

2. Ruptured ectopic pregnancy

Symptoms:
- Acute pain
- Signs of blood loss, eg pallor, tachycardia, fainting.

3. Ruptured ovarian cyst

Symptoms:
- Acute unilateral pain radiating to the back.

4. Salpingitis

Symptoms:
- High fever
- Pain and peritonism across whole abdomen or more commonly the iliac fossa.

5. Ovarian Cancer

Symptoms:
- Non-specific lower abdominal pain
- Palpable mass if advanced.

6. Urinary Tract Infection

Symptoms:
- Lower abdominal or iliac fossa pain

- Fever
- Dysuria
- Frequency.

Assessment:
Urine test and culture.

Haemorrhagic Colitis

Causes include: reaction to penicillin-related antibiotics.[17]

Symptoms:
- Passing of fresh blood per rectum with diarrhoea (compare colonic carcinoma).

Hernia (inguinal or femoral)

Symptoms:
- Pain accompanied by small bowel obstruction

Assessment:
Observation and palpation.

Inflammatory Bowel Disease (IBD)
Crohn's disease and ulcerative colitis, are often classified as Inflammatory Bowel Disease.

Symptoms:
- Iron deficiency anaemia
- Skin lesions eg erythema nodosum, pyoderma gangrenosum.

Assessment:
IBD patients will have an increase in faecal lactoferrin levels. This will not be present in IBS.

Note:
Patients with chronic amoebic colitis caused by parasites such as entamoeba histolytica have been misdiagnosed as IBD.

[17] *Journal of Gastroenterology and Hepatology,* 1998; 13: 1115-18.

Ischaemic Colitis
This is caused by thrombosis of the arterial supply to the left colon.

Symptoms:
- Abdominal pain
- Bloody diarrhoea.

Assessments:
X-ray and CT scan.

Pancreatic carcinoma

Symptoms:
- Malabsorption causing foul smelling stool
- Sudden weight loss.

Compare: Coeliac disease.

Peritonitis

Symptoms:
- High fever
- Pain
- Severe weakness.

Rectal mucosal prolapse
This is more likely in geriatric patients.

Symptoms:
- A sense of blockage is felt in the rectum, with rectal straining to pass the motion.

Sub-acute bowel obstruction

Symptoms:
- Distention and pain.

Thyrotoxicosis

Symptoms:
- Diarrhoea

- Weight loss
- Heat intolerance
- Anxiety
- Tachycardia.

Assessment:
Thyroid Function Test. If doubt remains, refer for free T3 & T4 test. A finger prick test kit is now available in Australia.[18]

Ulcerative Colitis

Symptoms:

The most common symptoms of ulcerative colitis are abdominal pain and bloody diarrhoea.

Patients may also experience:

- Anaemia
- Fatigue
- Weight loss
- Loss of appetite
- Rectal bleeding
- Loss of body fluids and nutrients
- Skin lesions
- Joint pain
- Growth failure (specifically in children).

About half of the people diagnosed with ulcerative colitis have mild symptoms. Others suffer frequent fevers, bloody diarrhoea, nausea, and severe abdominal cramps. Ulcerative colitis may also cause problems such as arthritis, inflammation of the eye, liver disease, and osteoporosis.

Assessment:
Stool sample may reveal white blood cells. Barium enema. Colonoscopy or sigmoidoscopy are the most accurate assessments.

---

[18] One supplier is Analytical Reference Laboratories: www.arlaus.com.au

Zollinger-Ellison Syndrome

A gastrinoma causing gastric hypersecretion and peptic ulceration.

Symptoms:
- Diarrhoea.

Shortlist of symptom differentials

Symptom	Possible Diagnosis
Rebound pain on palpation	Appendicitis
Pain relief when not moving	Peritoneal inflammation
Pain preceding vomiting	Appendicitis, intestinal obstruction
Pain concurrent with vomiting	Gastroenteritis
Obstipation with thin stools	Obstructing lesion of the colon
Bloody or mucous stool	Malignancy, colonic ischaemia, colitis, haemorrhoids
Increasing pain with guarding tenderness & fever	Diverticulitis, abscess, appendicitis
Faeces passing through vagina	Colo-vaginal fistula or malignancy

Chapter 3
The Treatment of Irritable Bowel Syndrome

Category 1: Intestinal Parasitosis...51
Category 2: Dysbiosis & Candida of the GIT...61
Category 3: Emotional...63
Category 4: Food Sensitivity...67
Category 5: 'Never well since'...69
Category 6: Hypochlorhydria & Gastro-Oesophageal Reflux...71
Category 7: Gallbladder Stasis...74
Category 8: Gastritis & Peptic Ulcer...75
Category 9: Post Viral...77
Category 10: Constipation...79
Category 11: Diarrhoea & Faecal Incontinence...80
Category 12: Diet & Lifestyle...82
Category 13: Bowel Nosodes...83
Category 14: Particular symptoms where no other cause...86
Category 15: Cellular Memory...87

Each category represents either (i) a specific cause of IBS and treatment recommendations for it, or (ii) offers a particular treatment option (without any clear causes) when no other category or cause of IBS can be found. A patient may need successive treatment from more than one category.

It is important for the patient to experience improvement of symptoms early in the treatment, so that he feels encouraged to persist with homeopathic treatment until symptom-free. The protocols described in this chapter are recommended to ensure rapid and steady improvement. Constitutional prescribing may also be necessary to bring the treatment to a conclusion.

Impediment to cure

If one opens a case with a constitutional medicine without first treating a pathology (eg parasites) or removing an impediment to cure (eg a 'never well since'), the constitutional medicine will not bring the patient to cure. This is because intestinal parasites and a 'never well since' causation are exogenous disease causations: they have entered the patient's *dynamis* from the external world. All the other categories of IBS are endogenous (they are an expression of the patient's vital force.) An exogenous disease phenomenon must be removed before constitutional prescribing is commenced. Unless first removed, it remains an impediment to cure. This is discussed in greater detail in Chapter 6.

Category 1: Intestinal Parasitosis

Most common causation of IBS
I have found in clinic that the presence of, or susceptibility to, intestinal parasites, causes all of the symptoms described in Chapter 1, including food sensitivities, increased allergic responses, disturbed sleep, abdominal pain and diarrhoea. Some 70 per cent of patients with IBS have intestinal parasitosis as part, or all, of the cause of their symptoms. It is therefore very effective to commence treatment in the majority of cases with one of the protocols for intestinal parasites described here.

From a homeopathic point of view, the precise pathogen is less important than the presenting symptoms. Allopathic treatment measures can be ineffective in these chronic cases because the susceptibility of the patient needs to be altered. Allopathic medicine may eradicate some or all of the pathogens, but unless the susceptibility of the patient is changed, symptoms will eventually return, despite the temporary relief being achieved. Homeopathic medicine can change the gut environment and dynamic sensitivity of the patient so that parasitic organisms no longer find the host a welcome home.

Symptoms in Intestinal Parasitosis:
Clinical experience shows that patients will have one or more of the following symptoms:

- Abdominal pain especially umbilical
- Allergies (including colds and flues)
- Anaemia
- Anorexia
- Anxiety*
- Bloating
- Constipation*
- Diarrhoea*
- Emaciation
- Fatigue
- Flatulence
- Flushes of heat
- Insomnia

- Irritability*
- Nasal itch*
- Nausea
- Night terrors*
- Nocturnal fever*
- Rectal itch*
- Restless leg syndrome
- Skin itch or crawling sensation
- Teeth grinding*
- Variable appetite*
- Weakness
- Weight loss

*These symptoms are commonly found in children

Children with ongoing diarrhoea, steatorrhoea and poor weight gain should of course be assessed for coeliac disease. The medicines and dosage recommendations for children are identical to those used for adults.

There are four significant medicines used to treat patients with intestinal parasites. The medicines are listed here from the most to the least commonly prescribed.

(a) *Cina* and *Stannum met* are used in the majority of cases.
(b) *Teucrium* is less often prescribed.
(c) When either of these medicines has improved that patient well, yet residual symptoms persist despite prolonged treatment (for many months in some cases), one should next use *Trichinose Nosode*. *Trichinose* can then produce a complete resolution of symptoms.

Cina

Medicines such as *Cina* are described in the *Materia Medicas* with reference to children. However, intestinal parasitosis is equally common among adults and is a major cause of IBS. The irritable child may need *Cina,* however there is another dimension to this medicine. My experience is that a patient treated with *Cina* may also experience improvement in anxiety. *Anxiety or irritability* are therefore appropriate keynotes for prescribing *Cina.* There may be insomnia, restless leg syndrome, teeth-grinding, rectal and nasal itch, in children or adults.

Patients requiring Cina have *diarrhoea, more often than constipation*, as part of their IBS symptom picture. A keynote for *Cina* would be agitation or irritability of the nervous system.

- *Cina 200*: One dose every second day for at least one month:
    - IBS symptoms +
    - *Emotional disturbance: irritability and/or anxiety*
    - Rectal, nasal or palate itching
    - Sinus symptoms in some cases, "allergies"
    - Teeth clenching
    - Disturbed sleep, including night terrors
    - Itching, prickly heat, or crawling skin sensations
    - Flushes of heat or actual fevers
    - Restless leg syndrome
    - Vomiting, diarrhoea and constipation.

Stannum Met
Stannum appears to display no particular mentals in parasitosis. The focus of symptoms is abdominal pain, which is particularly felt around the umbilicus. *Stannum* is alternated with *Nux vom 30* because the latter will improve peristalsis and help to reduce the abdominal pain; while *Stannum* focuses on changing the intestinal environment which is conducive to parasitosis. The *Materia Medica* for *Stannum* describes umbilical pain, which is the most common site for parasite-induced abdominal pain. Patients requiring *Nux vom* complain that they 'never feel completely empty' after passing their stool. Therefore, patients requiring *Stannum* and *Nux vom* have *constipation more often than diarrhoea*, as part of their IBS symptom picture.

In cases where diarrhoea is a prominent symptom *with* the umbilical pain, one can prescribe *Stannum met 200* every second day *without* the *Nux vom 30* on alternate days. *Nux vom* is unnecessary if there is complete bowel evacuation.

In *Stannum,* the irritability and anxiety are not prominent as in *Cina.* The focus of the symptoms is the abdominal pain, especially where it is around the umbilicus. That is not to say that these patients never experience anxiety, but it is more likely to be in the form of disturbing dreams (or night terrors in children). If anxiety is a *prominent* symptom in the patient's disturbance, *Cina* will yield a better result. Keynotes for *Stannum* would be 'sluggishness and pain'.

- *Stannum Met 200 & Nux vom 30*: One dose on alternate days for at least one month:
    - IBS symptoms +
    - *Abdominal pain especially around the umbilicus*
    - Constipation or never fully empty sensation when the bowels open
    - Sinus symptoms in some cases, "allergies"
    - Disturbed sleep including night terrors.

Teucrium
Although this is a small medicine in the treatment of intestinal parasitosis, it is nonetheless important where symptoms are focussed on the post-nasal and rectal area. *Teucrium* also displays no particular mental disturbance, but has a strong post-nasal symptomatology: with chronic post-nasal drip and/or clinkers. In some cases there are nasal polyps. Irritation of the nasal mucosa causes the patient to scratch the nose. Rectal itch is also found with this medicine.

Its other field of action is in adults or children who appear thin and emaciated, no matter how much they eat. Their appetite may be lacking. In these cases, *Teucrium* is a more appropriate prescription choice than *Cina*.

A keynote of *Teucrium* would be 'congestive nasal symptoms combined with emaciation'. Compare the Bowel nosode *Gaertner*, discussed later.

- *Teucrium 200*: One dose on alternate days for at least one month:
    - IBS symptoms +
    - *Chronic post nasal symptoms* with thick, purulent mucus
    - Rectal itch
    - Disturbed sleep including night terrors
    - Nasal polyps
    - Emaciation, weight loss, anaemia.

Trichinose Nosode[19]

Trichinose Nosode has similar mentals to *Cina.* It improves irritability or anxiety. *Trichinose* may be prescribed if one of the above medicines has worked well, but the case keeps relapsing. This will bring about complete removal of parasitic symptoms in many cases. It follows well after any of the above medicines when the following symptoms persist.

- *Trichinose Nosode 30:* One dose every second day for at least one month:
    - Diarrhoea
    - Abdominal pain with bloating after meals
    - Disturbed sleep
    - Anxiety or irritability
    - Teeth clenching
    - Headaches.

Pathology must be treated before a 'mentals' prescription

All four medicines above may show disturbance of sleep, which in children may be night terrors. In my experience, if one prescribes a medicine based on the mentals alone which does not take into account the presence of intestinal parasites, it will not be very effective. This is because it does not address the cause of the problem. For example, a patient has night terrors with fear to be alone in the dark. If this patient's emotional symptoms appear as a result of intestinal parasitosis, *Stramonium* will only have a temporary or incomplete effect. One of the above four medicines will be needed to cure the case, since *Stramonium* does not address the intestinal pathology.

Posology

The above medicines generally need repetition every second day for at least one month, during which time improvement is usually seen. Repetition should be continued every second day, or less often, provided improvement continues, sometimes for many months. Frequency of doses is slowly reduced provided improvement continues.

---

[19] Humans can contract trichiniasis from eating under-cooked meat. It causes diarrhoea and abdominal pain, nausea, periorbital oedema, myalgia, fever, headache. In rare cases there are neurologic and pulmonary complications. This nosode is available from selected homeopathic pharmacies.

A criticism of this approach is that long and frequent repetition of a medicine in the same potency may cause a 'proving' or aggravation of symptoms. I have not found this to be the case, especially where the patient experiences sustained relief for the first time in many years.

Aggravation
If aggravation occurs, it usually occurs at the start of treatment. On rare occasions, there is an aggravation for a few days to many weeks into the treatment, described by the patient as a 'catching a gastric bug'.

If one of the above medicines makes the patient worse, the cause is not intestinal parasites. 'Worse' should be clearly distinguished from 'aggravation'. When the patient aggravates, there will be a temporary aggravation of existing symptoms, lasting up to one week. If the medicine is making the patient worse, the worsening of symptoms will last for as long as the patient takes the medicine (ie over one week) and there *may be new symptoms appearing*. This is an indication from the vital force that the medicine selection is wrong. In these cases stop the medicine and revise your aetiology and diagnosis.

However, if an ongoing aggravation continues, then the medicine is incorrectly prescribed and another cause must be considered. Of course, the patient may not have IBS at all (refer to Chapter 2 for a differential diagnosis).

Suppression & Miasm
Another criticism of this approach is that the case is 'suppressed'. I do not believe this is the case for the following reason: the appropriately prescribed anti-parasitic medicine addresses the *cause* of the symptoms by *dynamically altering the patient's susceptibility* to intestinal parasitosis. This is confirmed when chronic IBS patients become symptom free. The parasitosis is a *concealed morbific influence* of the type that Hahnemann has described in *The Chronic Diseases*. The intestinal parasite is a chronic disease-producing agent, which causes systemic, functional disturbance, as well as local inflammation. In other words, one could describe parasitosis as a Chronic Miasm needing one of the anti-miasmatic medicines described here. In my opinion, parasitosis is precisely one of the

invisible *morbific* influences which Hahnemann first described. Medicines prescribed on the patient's symptoms may not treat the cause of those symptoms unless one uses an (anti-miasmatic) intestinal parasite medicine.

It is theoretical to suppose that this treatment is suppressive, since it is treating what is in essence a miasm. Accordingly, it is apt to describe patients in Category 1 of IBS, as having the Parasitic Miasm. This is discussed in more detail in Chapter 6.

Selecting the appropriate medicine

If symptoms are mixed and it is difficult to choose one of the above medicines, begin treatment with *Cina 200*, as described above. When in doubt, use *Cina.* Prescribe on the symptom or symptoms which are *worrying the patient the most.* For example, if a patient has regular umbilical pain with variable bowel habits, and this is the symptom which brought them in for consultation, even though there may also be some rectal itch, the disturbance to the patient is the *abdominal pain.* In this case, *Stannum* and *Nux vom* should be used in preference to *Cina* or *Teucrium.* If another patient has umbilical pain, plus great irritability or anxiety with diarrhoea, *Cina* is the preferred medicine, since the *emotional* symptoms are stronger. My observation is that long-term abdominal pain, especially if associated with parasitosis, produces profound emotional disturbance.

When no medicines work

The best selection of homeopathic medicines may fail to rid the patient of intestinal parasites, or fail to prevent immediate re-infection.

First, it is important that the above medicine of choice has been repeated every second day for at least one month. Improvement after one month will be apparent in most cases, after which the medicine should be continued until (i) all symptoms are resolved or (ii) new symptoms appear. Continue the medicine in *less frequent doses*, eg every third day, then every fourth day, etc. This may be continued for many months and should not be interrupted while the patient is improving.

If none of the above medicines has been effective, there are several possibilities:

i. This is not a case of intestinal parasitosis
ii. A different antiparasitic medicine to those above is required
iii. The patient has a pathology (eg coeliac disease)
iv. There is another cause of symptoms

(i) This is not a case of intestinal parasitosis
Refer to Chapter 2: Differential Diagnosis.

(ii) A different antiparasitic medicine is required
Here are some medicines which may be of value where the above medicines have not been effective:

- The patient is over-sensitive and impressionable. The body appears malnourished and there is a history of antibiotic use or gastroenteritis: the Bowel nosode *Gaertner 30 or 200.*

- Pain in the legs, headache, griping abdominal pain+++, possible squint, stammering, redness and irritation of the buccal mucosa with empty swallowing and palpitations. There may be a ravenous hunger combined with nausea and thirst: *Spigelia 200.*

- Intestinal parasitosis with recurrent fever: *Sulphur 200.*

- Hydatid cyst: *Thuja 30.*

- Umbilical pain and rectal itch are extreme and may result in convulsions: *Indigo 6.*

- Severe colic with foetid breath, salivation and severe hunger: *Mercurius sol 200.*

- *Cina-* type symptoms where the patient has not responded to either *Cina* or *Trichinose Nosode:* with symptoms affecting the bladder: *Terebinthina 200.*

- Sleepwalking associated with worms: *Artemisia vulg 1x.*

(iii) The patient has a pathology

If the patient has not yet been referred for colonoscopy or other pathology tests, now might be the time to do so.

(iv) There is another cause of symptoms (in addition to parasitosis)

Refer to Chapter 1: Diagnostic Criteria and Causes, and Chapter 2: Differential Diagnosis

Non-Homeopathic Treatment Options

There are allopathic and herbal medicines which have antiparasitic properties. The allopathic medications are often effective, however patients regularly suffer side effects: commonly nausea and headaches. Their effect on the liver may also be an issue in chronically sick patients.

Herbal medicines do not generally produce significant side effects and can be of value in reducing the severity of, and eradication of, some intestinal parasites. The following herbal medicines are frequently used to treat intestinal parasitosis:

- *Black walnut (Juglans nigra) fruit*
- *Wormwood (Artemesia annua)* (also of promising value in the treatment of malaria*)*
- *Thyme oil*
- *Cinnamon bark oil*
- *Spanish origanum oil*
- *Barberry (Berberis vulg)*
- *Grapefruit seed*
- *Garlic*
- *Pau D'Arco.*

However, neither herbal nor allopathic medicines will alter the constitutional receptivity of the host to parasitic infestation, so re-infestation is possible. I have found homeopathic medicine effective in both treatment of infestation, and prevention of re-infestation, provided the chosen anti-parasitic medicine is repeated for many months.

Mini-Repertory
For selection of Anti-Parasite Medicines

Symptom	**Homeopathic Medicine**
Abdominal pain (umbilical)	*Stannum & Nux*
Allergies (incl colds & flues)	*Cina, Stannum, Teucrium, Trichinose*
Anaemia	*Teucrium*
Anorexia	*Cina, Stannum, Teucrium, Trichinose*
Anxiety	*Cina*
Bloating & flatulence	*Cina, Stannum, Teucrium, Trichinose*
Constipation	*Stannum & Nux*
Diarrhoea	*Cina, Teucrium*
Emaciation	*Teucrium*
Fatigue	*Cina, Stannum, Teucrium, Trichinose*
Flushes of heat	*Cina*
Insomnia	*Cina*
Irritability	*Cina*
Nasal itch	*Cina, Teucrium*
Nasal polyp	*Teucrium*
Nausea	*Cina, Stannum, Teucrium, Trichinose*
Night terrors (child)	*Cina, Stannum, Teucrium, Trichinose*
Nocturnal fevers	*Cina, Stannum, Teucrium, Trichinose*
Rectal itch	*Cina, Teucrium*
Restless leg syndrome	*Cina*
Skin itch or crawling sensation	*Cina*
Teeth grinding	*Cina, Stannum, Teucrium, Trichinose*
Umbilical pain	*Stannum & Nux*
Weakness	*Cina, Stannum, Teucrium, Trichinose*
Weight loss	*Cina, Stannum, Teucrium, Trichinose*

Category 2: Dysbiosis & Candida of the GIT

Symptoms:

- Abdominal bloating and flatulence
- Sugar and carbohydrate craving and/or intolerance
- Mood swings
- History of vaginal thrush or vaginitis
- Fatigue.

Candidiasis of the GIT is commonly found in women who have a history of vaginal candida (monilia). Unlike intestinal parasites, Candida albicans is a normal organism found in the human gut which has proliferated to an unhealthy level, often because of overuse of antibiotics or prolonged use of the oral contraceptive pill. Dietary factors also influence candida overgrowth; among these are too many refined carbohydrates. Many patients present with symptoms which show a relationship between fluctuating blood sugar levels and candida overgrowth.

Candida symptoms are similar to hypoglycaemic symptoms, so careful casetaking is needed to differentiate them. If the patient has tiredness and dizziness, or headache more than two hours after eating with a craving for sugar, think first of disturbance in sugar metabolism, rather than candidiasis. If there is a history of vaginal candidiasis with leucorrhoea or itching, then candida is more likely. *Both syndromes may occur concurrently.*

Treatment for candida-generated IBS symptoms:

- *Candida Albicans 20M:* twice daily for 10 days, plus
- *Lycopodium 30:* one to three times daily, depending on the severity of the abdominal bloating and the sugar sensitivity.

To treat candida symptoms where the symptom focus is vaginal itching:

- *Kreosotum 200:* one dose every second day for two to four weeks.

Once the patient has improved on *Candida albicans 20M* give *Candida albicans 50M* twice daily for a further ten days, while reducing *Lycopodium* to once or twice daily or even less frequently depending on the symptoms. The patient should avoid sugar during treatment and only eat fruit with other solid food.

Regeneration of the normal gut flora can be aided by taking probiotics. Kefir yoghurt has a reputation for recolonising the gut and is better tolerated by those with mild dairy intolerance.[20] See also the section on Bowel nosodes at p 83. According to Paterson[21], the use of the Bowel Nosodes can also restore the gut flora balance, and this is consistent with our experience.

---

[20] http://users.sa.chariot.net.au/~dna/kefirpage.html

[21] Paterson, J, *The Bowel Nosodes,* B Jain Publishers, New Delhi, 1988, reprinted from *The British Homeopathic Journal*, Vol XL, No 3, July 1950

Category 3: Emotional

Symptoms:

- Symptoms are aggravated during stress
- Symptoms may be better during sleep
- Thinking about symptoms may worsen them.

Emotional disturbance invariably requires constitutional treatment. However, if intestinal parasites or candida albicans of the GIT are diagnosed, be sure to treat those pathologies *before* constitutional treatment. This will ensure an improvement resulting in greater patient and practitioner satisfaction. The treatment of emotional disturbance without removing gut pathology can result in incomplete treatment, or improvement which does not hold. This can be confusing, as emotional symptoms are often clouded by the presence of the gut pathology. If you suspect intestinal parasites are connected with emotional disturbance a course of *Cina 200,* as described above, will confirm or deny your suspicion. This will remove any obstacle to cure.

Since constitutional and 'mentals' prescriptions are highly individual selections, no potency or posology recommendations have been given below. However, here are some common medicines I have found work well for patients with IBS:

- *Asafoetida:* This is a major medicine for IBS with hysteria. The hysterical aspect is the keynote. Anxiety is experienced as a somatic sensation in the epigastrium or gut. The patient may be unable to tell whether his symptoms are anxiety or gut disturbance, since both have become enmeshed. Diarrhoea or constipation, with much flatulence. There is reflux with regurgitation and forcible burping. There are tight spasms or pulsations, always worse for anxiety.

- *Phosphorus:* Overly sensitive to others' emotions. Sensitive to non-physical phenomena (may be psychic), and particularly to dark, storms or 'evil' energies. History of nightmares,. Also sensitive to visual impressions or sounds, eg cannot watch horror films. There may be a history of sleepwalking. The gut symptoms are diarrhoea and pain which *exhaust* the patient. There is a weak, empty or all-gone sensation in the abdomen.

- *Colocynthis:* Severe spasmodic pains, worse after anger, irritation or becoming overly excited. The patient may be easily angered. Pains are ameliorated from bending forward or from firm pressure on the abdomen.

- *Nux vom:* Pain around the umbilical ring. Retro-sternal pain in reflux or hiatus hernia. The patient is typically chilly, easily angered, overworked. He is fastidious, competitive and impatient.

- *Chamomilla:* The patient is beside himself with the pain and consequently does not want to be touched. The *Chamomilla* child is typically capricious, irritable, and inconsolable owing to the effect of the pain on him.

- *Ignatia:* Symptoms are contradictory or do not add up. The patient may have quick mood swings and is easily moved to tears. The emotions feel out of control. Anxiety is easily somaticised into the abdomen or the throat, causing tightness and a sense of weight. The patient may be on the verge of tears. Along with *Asafoetida, Ignatia* is one of the most hysterical medicines.

- *Cina:* This medicine is described in detail under Category 1 at p 52.

- *Argentum nit:* Anticipatory anxiety with great fear of enclosed spaces. Diarrhoea occurs before anticipated events. Loud eructations, abdominal distension and rumbling. Aggravation from sweets.

- *Lycopodium:* This is the best polychrest for flatulence and bloating, regardless of the patient's mentals. However, in classic *Lycopodium* patients there is low self-esteem, whose compensation is irritability, especially at home. They need to 'keep up appearances', such as over-preparing work so that it cannot be faulted. Typically the patient is critical, does not tolerate fools, is somewhat egotistical and intellectual. Aggravation on right side, at 4 to 8 pm, and from sugar.

- *Arsenicum:* Anxious, fastidious, competitive, obsessive, chilly. History of insomnia. Diarrhoea and vomiting. Aggravation after eating. Pains are burning in nature. Use *Arsenicum 3* if treating peptic ulcer or severe gastritis: see p 76. *Arsenicum 3* is not recommended in peptic ulcer with haematemesis.

- *Carcinosin:* History of insomnia, extremely fastidious and anxious. Family history of cancer or diabetes. Never well since glandular fever. History of childhood infectious diseases as an adult. Ameliorated by the sea, storms. Sensitive to reprimand.

- *Stramonium:* Fears being alone in the dark, either in reality or in the dreams. A history of being exposed to violence, or of having terror of the likelihood of violence to oneself.

- *Calcarea phos:* Psychosomatic abdominal pain in children or teenagers, with or without headaches. Desire for salt and smoked food. Growing pains. Typically, the child is peevish or discontented.

- *Causticum:* Patients whose symptoms can manifest after a strong empathic experience. Intolerant of injustice. There may be a foreboding that something bad will happen, though the patient may not know what. Aggravation from winds. Desires salt and smoked food.

- *Natrum mur:* The patient has a history of grief, such that when recalling the event many years later, s/he cries as if it were recent. Feels s/he is an outsider and lives in an inner world where no one else may travel. Desire for salt.

- *Opium:* When recalling a specific shock, the patient still experiences anxiety at the memory. This is described in the *Repertory* as 'fear of the fright'.

- *Phosphoric ac:* Either long-standing grief, or diarrhoea, have produced a deep indifference in the patient. The patient presents as depressed.

- *Carbo veg:* All foods appear to aggravate the patient: everything turns into eructation or flatulence. The patient loses vitality owing to the long-standing nature of the illness, and may never have fully recovered from a previous illness.

- *Mercurius sol:* Diarrhoea with a mucous discharge. The patient is typically suspicious and is given to compulsive, sometimes violent, impulses which s/he works hard to constrain. Aggravation at night.

Rubrics for IBS with emotional disturbance
These medicines have strong bowel symptoms in their *Materia Medica*:

- Ailments from anger: *Colocynthis, Nux vom, Chamomilla, Ignatia, Cina, Opium.*

- Ailments from anxiety: *Argentum nit, Lycopodium, Arsenicum, Carcinosin, Phosphorus, Stramonium, Ignatia.*

- Ailments from grief: *Calcarea phos, Causticum, Ignatia, Natrum mur, Nux vom, Opium, Phosphorus, Phosphoric ac.*

- Ailments from guilt: *Arsenicum, Carbo veg, Causticum, Ignatia, Mercurius, Natrum mur, Nux vom, Phosphoric ac.*

- Hysterical gastro-intestinal symptoms: *Asafoetida, Ignatia, Argentum nit, Cina.*

Category 4: Food Sensitivity

Symptoms:

- Aggravation of symptoms following a certain food or group of foods.

Many cases of apparent food sensitivity disappear when parasitosis is successfully treated as described in Category 1, p 52. Similarly, treating hypochlorhydria, gallbladder stasis and candidiasis can also improve food sensitivities. It is always beneficial for the patient to refrain from foods which aggravate his symptoms until the underlying causes have been significantly addressed by the appropriate protocol. The most common of these food sensitivities are:

- Wheat and gluten
- Cow's milk products
- Yeast
- Salicylates
- Eggs
- Peanuts.

Even after successful treatment of IBS the food sensitivities may not disappear altogether. The patient may still need to refrain from, or have minimal amounts of, the offending foods. Prolonged abstinence can remove the sensitivity.

During the abstaining period measures to restore normal gut flora should be taken. Patients sometimes respond to an isopathic preparation of the offending food, for example:

- *Wheat 12:* one dose daily for two weeks; followed by
- *Wheat 6:* one dose daily for two weeks.

A challenge after this desensitising protocol may reveal significant improvement in the sensitivity. It is not recommended to try this desensitisation if the patient has coeliac disease. The best treatment for coeliac disease remains strict avoidance of gluten.

As well as avoiding offending foods in the short term, appropriate eating habits are important. Many people have a carbohydrate dominant diet, resulting in hypoglycaemic episodes. These patients must be encouraged to eat protein with their carbohydrates, and chew their food well.

General dietary considerations:

- Decrease coffee, tea and alcohol consumption
- Decrease sugar and refined carbohydrates
- Small, regular meals each containing protein
- Avoid overeating or undereating
- Make sure the diet has enough fresh fruit, vegetables and nuts
- Maintain adequate intake of mineral or spring water
- Take probiotics at night or kefir to normalize gut flora.

Category 5: 'Never Well Since'

A 'never well since' (NWS) aetiology takes treatment priority over constitutional prescribing. The effectiveness of the latter will be diminished if the 'never well since' (NWS) obstacle is not first removed. Some 'never well since' obstacles are described below.

Symptoms:

- There are no symptoms specific to this category. Diagnosis will be made solely from the patient's history, when the onset of symptoms follows a specific illness or event.

NWS Antibiotics with IBS symptoms

If the patient has IBS plus non-GIT symptoms, such as sinusitis, ever since taking antibiotics, the tautopathic approach described below is very effective.

- *Penicillin or Amoxicillin 30:* One dose daily for five to 10 days. Patients often experience aggravation of symptoms when taking these tautopathic medicines. This usually passes within one to three days, followed by the removal of symptoms. Use this treatment where patients date the origin of their symptoms to the use of antibiotics. However, *if those antibiotics were used to treat gastroenteritis, it is likely that the subsequent IBS was caused by the gastroenteritic pathogen, not the antibiotics, in which case one of the treatment protocols for intestinal parasites should be chosen.*

- *Gaertner 30:* This medicine can work well in treating post-antibiotic symptoms. Consider this Bowel nosode when well-selected medicines fail.

NWS Glandular Fever (Infectious Mononucleosis) with IBS symptoms

- *Coxsackievirus 30:* One dose every second day for up to one month. *Coxsackie* is a very effective medicine for rapidly removing the sequelae of glandular fever, with minimal aggravation. The patient may report no history of glandular fever, but their spouse has had the disease. Even though no acute symptoms were experienced by the patient, intimate communication with someone who has had the virus may transmit a symptom phenomenon, the precise nature of which is thus far unclear. There is an unexplained phenomenon in which carers of CFS sufferers could develop similar symptoms to their patients. Please see further Post Viral at p 77. See also Case 6, p 10.8 If *Coxsackievirus* is ineffective consider one of the following:

- *Carcinosin 30 or 200:* One dose every second day. The patient has insomnia, anxiety with fastidiousness.
- *Glandular Fever Nosode 1M:* A single dose can bring about relief of symptoms, however this remedy can cause severe aggravation, so *Coxsackievirus* should first be given.

NWS Abdominal surgery

- *China 6:* Incarcerated flatus after surgery; or passing wind affords no relief of the abdominal distention and discomfort.
- *Staphysagria 200:* Systemic symptoms, including those other than gastrointestinal, which appear since the surgery.
- *Allium*-c 30: Thread-like pain remaining at the site of the surgical wound.

NWS Other diseases

- *Carbo veg 200:* A generalised state of weakness persists with tremendous bloating and indigestion after almost any food. ('I don't know what to eat'). The patient feels better after burping or passing flatus. Moist stools or diarrhoea, foul smelling and sometimes with mucus.

NWS Use of Oral Contraceptive Pill (OCP)

- *Folliculinum 30:* One dose every second day. The patient should discontinue the OCP if it is still being used and use an alternative form of contraception. See Case 11 in Chapter 4.

NWS Other Allopathic Medication

- There are many allopathic medications which cause diarrhoea. This effect can be stopped by taking *Camphor 200,* twice daily for at least one week. If a patient is taking essential allopathic medication concurrently with *Camphor,* take care as it may completely antidote the therapeutic effect of that medication.

Category 6: Hypochlorhydria & Gastro-Oesophageal Reflux

Symptoms:

- IBS symptoms as described above +
- Sharp or burning pain (heartburn) felt at the cardiac orifice, oesophagus, trachea or larynx
- Dysphagia
- Voice loss or croaky voice
- Regurgitation and/or excessive burping
- Sensation of tightness around the throat
- Abdominal bloating

A Pathogenic Cause of Gastric Reflux

It is widely acknowledged that there is a pathogenic cause of peptic ulcer: helicobacter pylori. Is it possible that other gastric symptoms may have a pathogenic cause? Some IBS patients also experience reflux. Could that reflux be caused by the same intestinal parasites which I have suggested cause IBS? Early clinical evidence suggests this might be probable in a small number of cases, whose reflux symptoms show improvement once intestinal parasites are treated. This is examined in more detail in Chapter 6.

However, most patients treated for parasitosis will require a different homeopathic medicine for their reflux.

Hypochlorhydria

As stated elsewhere [22], hypochlorhydria is a common yet unacknowledged cause of gastric reflux. Low stomach hydrochloric acid is more common than hyperchlorhydria (excessive stomach hydrochloric acid).

Non-Homeopathic Treatment

The treatment of hypochlorhydria necessitates a diet which will stimulate hydrochloric acid (HCl), even where there is gastritis or dyspepsia. Patients may think that stimulation of their stomach acid is the wrong approach, since they have been told for years that they

---

[22] Gamble, J, *Mastering Homeopathy: Accurate Daily Prescribing for a Successful Practice,* Karuna Publishing, Wollongong, Australia, 2004

have too much acid. Unfortunately, their treatment, which normally consists of a medication to suppress HCl, may have managed, but has not improved, the condition, since as soon as the patient reduces the medication, symptoms return immediately.

Patients should be instructed to avoid bland diets. Any of the aromatic culinary herbs, ie curries with turmeric, cardamom, cumin etc, will stimulate HCl. A small amount of hot chili can be homeopathic, but use with caution, especially in the case of gastric ulcer, as it may aggravate if taken in too large a quantity. If a small amount can be tolerated, it should be encouraged. The patient should avoid liquids before, during and immediately after meals, as this further dilutes the HCl.

To treat hypochlorhydria:

- *Gentian MT:* Mother tincture of *Gentian*, 15 to 20 drops in a little water, 20 minutes before each meal. If this causes heartburn, take it immediately before meals until it no longer causes heartburn, then return slowly to the 20 minute gap. Alternatively, add more water to the mixture.

Poor bile flow / Gallbladder stasis

In many cases of stomach acid disturbance, especially where diet has been particularly poor, the bile flow is inadequate to properly digest fats, resulting in reflux and bloating. The patient may experience:

- Pale stools
- Nausea
- Afternoon headaches
- Fatty food intolerance.

In these cases, to stimulate bile flow:

- *Chelidonium MT:* 15-20 drops of the mother tincture in water 20 minutes before each meal. *Chelidonium* can be mixed together with *Gentian*. The dose in these cases is 20-25 drops of the combined tinctures, as described. If the patient experiences pain in the epigastrium or the right hypochondrium when taking *Chelidonium* tincture, it is likely that there are gallbladder calculi. The patient should discontinue Chelidonium and have an ultrasound to check for calculi.

For further discussion of gastric reflux, see 'Gastritis & Peptic Ulcer' at p 75 and Gallbladder stasis at p 74.

Category 7: Gallbladder Stasis

Symptoms:

- Pale stools
- Nausea
- Afternoon headaches
- Fatty food intolerance
- Dull epigastric pain
- Dull right pain in the right hypochondrium.

Sludge of the bile duct is a not uncommon cause of these symptoms, as is gallbladder calculi. Unlike calculi, sludge is not evident on ultrasound, and is best diagnosed on the presenting symptoms listed above. Gallbladder stasis is usually a concomitant factor, not a sole cause, of IBS.

Treatment of gallbladder sludge:

- *Chelidonium tincture:* 15-20 drops of the mother tincture in water 20 minutes before each meal, for at least four weeks. If the patient experiences pain in the epigastrium or the right hypochondrium when taking *Chelidonium* tincture, it is likely that there are gallbladder calculi. Discontinue *Chelidonium* and refer for ultrasound.

Category 8: Gastritis & Peptic Ulcer

Symptoms:

- IBS symptoms as described above +
- Heartburn (sharp or burning pain) felt at cardiac orifice, epigastrium, oesophagus, trachea or larynx
- Dysphagia
- Voice loss or croaky voice
- Cough and/or mucus in the larynx, sometimes rising to the posterior nares
- Regurgitation and/or excessive burping with or without pain
- Sensation of tightness or lump in the throat
- Bloating.

Some IBS patients also experience reflux as part of their IBS picture. If treating intestinal parasites brings on improvement and will require one or more of the treatments below:

Gastritis with reflux:

- *Robinia 3:* Heartburn and reflux where the burning sensation extends from the stomach, up to the oesophagus. Sour burping. The pain occurs some time after eating. *Robinia* can be mixed with *Nat phos 3x* for better results. In chronic cases, this can be repeated for months.

- *Asafoetida 30:* Hysteria is the keynote. Reflux with regurgitation and forcible burping. There are tight spasms always worse for anxiety. The patient's symptoms are worse, or come on, when he thinks of them. Anxiety is experienced as a somatic sensation always felt in the epigastrium or gut. The patient may be unable to tell whether the symptoms are anxiety or gut disturbance, since the two can become enmeshed.

- *Abies nig 6:* A sensation of a lump in the top of the stomach (ie cardiac orifice) 'as if he had swallowed an egg'.

- *Arsenicum 3:* Severe epigastric pain immediately after eating, with vomiting which then relieves the pain. Do not use *Arsenicum* if there is haematemesis.

- *Lycopodium 30:* Abundant flatulence. The flatus may cause reflux because of the pressure it places on the stomach and pylorus.

- *Ignatia 200:* Reflux with minimal or no pain: there is merely a sensation of a lump in the throat, or sometimes a scratchy larynx. In other cases there is a specific small, sharp, constant pain retro-sternally. The patient is often anxious, however this symptom is not essential for the successful use of *Ignatia.*

Gastritis without Reflux:

- *Chelidonium 30:* Poor appetite and epigastric pain, yet the pain is improved by eating. Pain in the right hypochondrium, radiating to the right scapula (compare gallbladder calculi).

- *Anacardium 200:* Where there is a good appetite and the epigastric or hypochondrial pain is also improved by eating.

- *Arsenicum 3:* Can also be used for epigastric pain, where there is no reflux. Aggravation occurs immediately after food, which is relieved by vomiting.

- *Iris vers 200*: A burning pain is experienced *only* in the epigastric region, with no pain radiating up into the oesophagus.

Peptic Ulcer:

Ulceration can be treated with any of the above remedies, depending on the presenting symptoms. The most common, and successful, prescription is:

- *Arsenicum 3* alternated with *Anacardium 200:* One dose of either medicine on alternate days. Patients usually report improvement within two weeks.

Category 9: Post Viral

Symptoms:

- IBS symptoms as described +
- Fatigue
- Nausea
- Repeated colds, flues or throat infections (= lowered immunity)
- Clear onset of symptoms with a virus
- Ongoing cyclic diarrhoea or abdominal cramps
- Migraine
- Unexplained myalgia.

There is a small group of cases whose IBS symptoms appear to be post-viral. This is a hitherto unrecognised cause of IBS. The Epstein-Barr virus, cytomegalovirus, or similar type viruses, may lead to these unusual IBS cases.

IBS symptoms have a cyclic, acute onset. Their symptoms may appear, for example, once per month, and last for many days to one or two weeks. They are largely free of bowel symptoms between attacks, yet they complain of a general feeling of being unwell, described as excessive fatigue, or vague nausea. The acute attacks may consist of severe abdominal cramps and diarrhoea. These symptoms might lead one to assume they have an amoebic parasitic infection, such as giardia or cryptosporidium. However, when given the medicines already described to treat these pathogens (eg *Cina, Stannum, Teucrium*), there is no improvement, or an aggravation without improvement, results.

Patients with post-viral IBS have been exposed to a virus such as Epstein-Barr (the pathogen implicated in infectious mononucleosis or glandular fever); yet they may not have experienced any of the acute symptoms of that disease, such as pharyngitis and tonsillitis. They may have had exposure to the virus through a partner and not have ever developed symptoms of infectious mononucleosis.

- *Coxsackievirus 30:* One dose every second day for at least one month.

This medicine may produce a small aggravation each time it is taken, such as a vague sore throat, nausea or fatigue, followed by rapid improvement. I find that whenever the patient complains of being unwell since exposure to the Epstein-Barr or similar virus, *Coxsackievirus* is one of the best medicines for prompt improvement or outright cure.

While it is possible that IBS presents as one part of Chronic Fatigue Syndrome, the above symptoms are not CFS without the typical markers for that disease as I have described elsewhere.[23]

These patients will often improve with the use of a Bowel nosode, such one of the Morgan types prescribed on presenting symptomatology. However, cure is more likely with the use of the *Coxsackievirus,* which will become a major treatment of post-viral syndromes as it becomes more recognised.

---

[23] Gamble, J, *Mastering Homeopathy: Accurate Daily Prescribing for a Successful Practice,* Karuna Publishing, Wollongong, Australia, 2004

Category 10: Constipation

Symptoms:

- Less than one bowel motion per day
- No urge for stool
- Ineffectual urging for stool.
- Constipation with overflow symptoms, where small amounts of loose stool are passed, which present as 'diarrhoea'.

Overuse of laxatives and lack of dietary bulk (fibre) can cause a 'lazy' bowel, with inadequate peristalsis and muscle spasm. Constipation-dominant IBS can also be caused by intestinal parasites. It should be remembered that there are numerous causes of constipation, which include a host of allopathic medications (ie iatrogenic cause), anxiety over toileting, lifestyle factors, and endocrine disorders: see Chapter 1 at pp 32-33 for a complete list. Heavy metal toxicity may be present, which can be revealed by a hair mineral analysis.

Treatment of constipation-dominant IBS:

- *Bryonia 200:* The best medicine for long-standing constipation, when used in the 200th potency for optimum effect, and repeated initially every second day. The stool is large, hard and dry. The patient may experience pain in the right hypochondrium.

- *Plumbum 200:* This medicine can be alternated with *Bryonia* on alternate days if there is insufficient response with the latter prescribed alone. *Plumbum* is particularly useful in treating the elderly.

- *Nux vom 30:* The patient reports a 'never completely satisfied' feeling, even though a stool may be passed several times each day.

- *Alumina 200:* The preferred medicine in extremes of age where the stool is soft yet difficult to pass.

Category 11: Diarrhoea & Faecal Incontinence

A major cause of IBS with diarrhoea is intestinal parasitosis. If you deem this not to be the case, the medicines below need to be considered.

Inappropriate diet or food sensitivity may predispose to diarrhoea, with or without pain. While increased dietary fibre is often recommended, too much dietary fibre in some patients may be one reason for unexplained diarrhoea. An inability to tolerate dietary fibre is diagnostic of gut dysbiosis.

Patients with loose stools may have constipation with overflow. If small amounts are passed regularly but satisfactory bowel motions are seldom achieved, the patient is likely to be constipated.

Symptoms:

- Unformed or partially formed, urgent stool.

Other causes of faecal incontinence:

- Congenital
- Obstetric trauma
- Neurological disease
- Rectal prolapse
- Post-colon and rectal surgery or other iatrogenic trauma to anal sphincter
- Spinal trauma.

Specific medicines to treat diarrhoea:

- *Aloe 200:* Faecal incontinence. The patient is unsure if he is passing flatulence or stool which can lead to faecal accidents. Give one dose every second day.

- *Podophyllum 200:* Loose, watery stools with rumbling abdomen and slight pain.

- *Mercurius cor 30:* Diarrhoea with abdominal cramps, possibly some mucus or blood (colonic investigation may be required).

- *Colocynthis 200:* Diarrhoea with severe abdominal cramps causing the patient to bend over double. There is amelioration from pressure or assuming the foetal position. In one case where *Colocynthis* was effective, the spasms were so severe as to cause the patient to double up involuntarily.

Category 12: Diet & Lifestyle

The best homeopathic medicine will not undo an obstacle to cure such as poor diet. Skipping meals and reliance on convenience food can result in inadequate nutrition and disturbance to bowel habits. Taking vitamins may assist with nutritional deficiencies, but a diet which does not include fresh food is not conducive to physical or mental health.

Therefore, inappropriate lifestyle habits must be considered before prescribing any medicine. Failure to do so means an obstacle to cure is missed. The use of regular recreational drugs or an inappropriate working environment can cause symptoms. Chilly people do not tolerate air-conditioned offices well. A person prone to insomnia should not work night shifts and requires a regulated sleeping routine. Either of these scenarios can lead to poor health.

Large, infrequent meals may put significant pressure on the digestive system, and are a possible factor in indigestion and reflux. Similarly, under-eating, if severe, may lead to poor nutrition, disturbance to metabolism and energy, and may be a result of, or lead to, psychological disorders such as anorexia.

Given the extent of dietary error and stressful lifestyles, patients often improve by correcting their diet. If the addition of dietary fibre is going to be tried, this should be done for at least one week before its effectiveness is assessed.

Lifestyle factors may include:

- Excessive use of caffeine
- Inadequate water intake
- Inadequate sleep
- Long working hours
- Poor nutrition
- Lack of exercise
- Eating meals too quickly (thus swallowing air)
- Irregular shift work preventing bowel habits becoming regular.

Other Treatment Options

Category 13: Bowel Nosodes of Bach & Paterson[24]

Symptoms:

- IBS + other body systems affected
- IBS + emotional disturbance
- IBS where well-selected remedies have failed.

The Bowel nosodes are very potent medicines in the treatment of IBS, allergies, and symptom pictures where the gut is affecting other body systems or in cases where there is emotional disturbance with the IBS. Bowel nosodes are particularly relevant where the patient experiences many systemic symptoms in addition to IBS. This may include airborne allergies and hypersensitivity reactions. Bowel nosodes may also be used where the patient does not fit into any of the above categories, or where medicines suggested in those categories have not been effective. These nosodes can be given as an outright treatment or as an intercurrent medicine, after which one can return to the medicine of choice.

- *Gaertner*: This medicine can be used as a specific for the after-effects of antibiotics, irrespective of the constitution. As a result, it is useful for gut dysbiosis and leaky gut syndrome caused either by antibiotics or other factors. Experience lends support to this idea, particularly if *Penicillin* has been given in potency and not yielded a satisfactory response. The *Gaertner* patient may be oversensitive, with many fears. One can place this patient somewhere between a *Phosphorus* and *Silicea* type. There may be a history of diarrhoea, malabsorption and weight loss.

[24] Paterson, J, *The Bowel Nosodes,* B Jain Publishers, New Delhi, 1988, reprinted from *The British Homeopathic Journal*, Vol XL, No 3, July 1950

- *Proteus*: The keynote for this medicine is *prolonged nervous tension.* This may produce either temper tantrums in a child or anxiety attacks, both of which tend to come on suddenly. If there are pains, they will also appear without warning and will tend to be spasmodic. Medicine relations are: *Ignatia* and *Nux vomica.*

- *Dysentery Co*: The keynote for this medicine is anticipatory anxiety. The anxiety, as with *Proteus,* has a marked effect on the nervous and gastro-intestinal symptoms, causing functional projectile vomiting in children, diarrhoea and regurgitation. The principal medicine relation is *Argentum nit.*

- *Morgan group*: Introspection, depression, combined with congestion. There are constipation, catarrh and skin affectations. Nauseous or bilious conditions suggest the use of this nosode. Note the sub-types of this medicine: *Morgan Gaertner & Morgan Pure.* The principal medicine relations are: *Calcarea Carb, Sulphur* and *Lycopodium.*

- *Sycotic Co:* A keynote for this medicine is irritability. It is of course a medicine for treatment of the Sycotic Miasm: thus the patient may have chronic catarrh, skin overgrowths and aggravation from damp. Medicine relation: *Natrum sulph.*

- *Bacillus No 7:* I have found this medicine useful where the keynote symptom is fatigue. The patient will wake tired after a good sleep and may have post-exertion malaise or tenderness. The medicine can thus be considered for those who are walking the path towards Chronic Fatigue Syndrome, *provided there are concomitant gut symptoms.* It is unlikely this medicine will effectively treat post-viral CFS, for which other medicines are recommended.[25]

---

[25] Gamble, J, *Mastering Homeopathy: Accurate Daily Prescribing for a Successful Practice,* Karuna Publishing, Australia, 2004, p 81

Bowel Nosodes: Key words for selection

Alternation of symptoms	*Mutabile*
Anticipatory anxiety	*Dysentery Co*
Asthma alternates with eczema	*Mutabile*
Avoids company	*Morgan (Bach); Morgan Pure*
Congestion & sluggishness	*Morgan (Bach)*
Criticism, highly sensitive to	*Dysentery Co*
Depressive	*Morgan (Bach)*
Eczema in children	*Morgan (Bach)*
Emaciation & malnutrition	*Gaertner (Bach)*
Fatigue – feels unfit for the task	*Bacillus #7*
Fidgety, shy	*Dysentery Co*
Hypersensitive: brain overactive	*Gaertner (Bach)*
Hysteria	*Proteus (Bach)*
Introspection	*Morg (Bach)*
Irritability	*Sycotic Co*
Nerve strain – brain storm (tantrums)	*Proteus (Bach)*
Spasm – neurological	*Proteus (Bach)*
Sudden onset	*Proteus (Bach)*
Violent outburst with kicking & screaming - tantrums	*Proteus (Bach)*

Category 14: Particular symptoms where no other cause is ascertained

These medicines will relieve the particular symptoms and may cure the patient if the symptom picture is exact.

- *Mercurius cor 30*: Abdominal pain with diarrhoea without evident mental symptoms or other aetiology. There may be mucus or blood with the stool (compare Crohn's disease and colitis).

- *Nux vom 30*: Pain associated with incomplete evacuation or 'never quite satisfied' feeling. Pain is usually felt around the umbilical area.

- *Colocynthis 200*: Sharp, severe pain causing patient to bend double and ameliorated by pressure on abdomen or assuming the foetal position.

- *Aloe 200*: Diarrhoea with slight pain associated with faecal incontinence ('not sure if passing stool or only flatus').

- *Plumbum 200*: Constipation with contractive pain as though the abdominal wall were pulled back to the spine by a string, or the rectum feels drawn upwards.

- *Lycopodium 30:* One of the best medicines for bloating and flatulence in any part of the abdomen.

- *Bryonia 200:* Pain in the right hypochondrium associated with long-standing constipation.

- *Ipecac 200:* Diarrhoea, sometimes with mucus, with pain in the left iliac fossa.

Category 15: Cellular Memory

My current thinking is that where a patient has been treated for intestinal parasites yet their symptoms persist in the same or altered form, this may be a cellular memory of the chronic disease which has become established in the nervous system.

The nerves in the bowel wall are so used to responding to the chronic inflammation or parasitic infection that they are reacting *as though the parasitic infection is still present.*

Similarly, where there has been trauma of any kind experienced in the gut, I suspect it is possible for the memory of it to manifest symptoms as though the trauma were still present. The kinds of trauma I am referring to are:

- Previous surgery or injury to the bowel
- Abdominal pain or spasm as a result of emotional trauma, which is re-experienced whenever the memory of that trauma is revisited or triggered.

In these cases I believe one needs a neurological medicine – not a gastrointestinal one – to resolve the symptoms. The nervous system is behaving as though the pathogen or trauma is still present. The medicine needed will be based on the mentals, generals and particulars of the patient. Its effect will be to 'short circuit' the memory retained in the nervous system.

This seems to be restating the need for an 'emotional' or constitutional medicine. The difference here is that there is a specific disease causation mingled with the emotional/constitutional aspects.

The following is a shortlist of medicines which may be needed. Please note that this list is not exhaustive. The practitioner should remember that the indicated medicine must have a neurological effect in its proving symptoms.

Shortlist of Medicines
Potency suggestions have only been given where a specific one has been found particularly efficacious. Give the medicine once every second day (unless you choose a high potency) until symptoms are resolved.

- *Ignatia 200:* Ongoing anxiety felt in the abdomen, oesophagus or trachea. The symptoms are worse when thinking about them. There may be griping abdominal pain with constricting spasm of the rectum after stool. IBS with gastric reflux.

- *Proteus 30 (Bowel nosode):* There is a sudden onset of a painful colonic spasm. The patient does not hold up well to stress.

- *Gaertner 30 (Bowel nosode):* Oversensitive, refined people (*Phos, Sil*) who may over-react to their bowel symptoms, thinking the worst. There is a long history of diarrhoea.

- *Morgan Bach (Bowel nosode):* Constipation. The patient may be depressed and withdrawn. The keynote is congestion.

- *Hyoscyamus 6:* The patient starts up from sleep. There are spasms and abdominal distention.

- *Spigelia 200:* Abdominal pain with sharp, griping, neuralgic-type pain. There may be history of stammering, rectal itch, offensive breath, inflamed pharynx or palpitations. Children may have ravenous hunger with thirst and nausea concomitants.

- *Carcinosin:* This medicine will suit the spastic colon patients whose symptoms are aggravated by their anxiety. The patient is fastidious, often anxious, with a history of insomnia and a family history of malignancy or diabetes. Adults may have experienced infectious childhood diseases. There is a lack of self confidence and a strong work focus. There is anticipatory anxiety and a strong desire to please others. Also consider: *Carcinosin-cum-cuprum.*[26]

---

[26] See Smits, Tinus, *Inspiring Homeopathy: the Treatment of Universal Layers,* 1999

- *Cuprum met 6:* Spasmodic, cramping pain. There may be reflux with vomiting relieved by drinking cold water. Hiccough may precede the spasms.

- *Asafoetida 6 or 30:* The keynote is the hysterical component. The patient's symptoms are worse, or come on, when he thinks of them. Anxiety is experienced as a sensation always felt in the epigastrium or gut. Diarrhoea or constipation, with much flatulence. There is reflux with regurgitation and forcibly burping. There are tight spasms always worse for anxiety. The patient may be unable to tell whether his symptoms are anxiety or gut disturbance, since the two become enmeshed.

- *Opium:* Recalling an emotional trauma brings on the abdominal symptoms, even though the original trauma has long passed, indicates *Opium* in high potency which will, as it were, unplug the link between the past event and the fear of it housed in one's memory. In the *Synthetic Repertory* this is referred to as 'Anxiety, fright, if fear or fright remain'. In Kent's *Repertory* it is called 'Anxiety, with fear of the fright'.

- *Staphysagria:* Use this medicine where the patient's symptoms date from abdominal surgery.

- *Allium c:* If there is a fine, thread-like pain remaining at the site of surgical trauma, *Allium* is a more precise prescription than *Staphysagria.*

Chapter 4
Cases

These cases are presented to illustrate the way I have used the treatment protocols described in this book.

Please note: all names in the following cases have been changed.

Case 1: Parasitosis with Anxiety and Insomnia ...92
Case 2: Iatrogenic IBS...96
Case 3: A Puzzling Case...99
Case 4: Parasitosis in Children...104
Case 5: Parasitosis and Gallbladder...106
Case 6: 'Never Well Since' and Post-viral...108
Case 7: Constipation...112
Case 8: Anxiety-related IBS...114
Case 9: Post-enteritis Parasitosis...117
Case 10: Chronic Sinusitis with IBS...120
Case 11: Emotional and Behavioural...123
Case 12: A Complex, Multi-Layered Case...126
Case 13: Parasitosis, Sinusitis and Chronic Anxiety...132

Case 1: Parasitosis with Anxiety and Insomnia

This is a case where I first observed a relationship between parasitosis, anxiety and insomnia.

Ann, Female, 30, presented with these symptoms:
Irritable bowel syndrome in excess of seven years. Severe stomach cramps after eating followed by diarrhoea lasting for one or two hours. She may be woken in the night with diarrhoea. Aggravation: fatty food; Chinese food; spicy food. The patient presents as a forthright, slightly anxious woman, with a busy lifestyle and one small child.

History
Migraine headaches every ten days.
Recurrent colds.
Several bouts of 'food poisoning'.
Allergy to bee stings.
Some food sensitivity to salicylates.

Particulars
Migraine headaches every 10 days, better during pregnancy and breastfeeding.
Grinding teeth.
Constant perspiration under arms.
Hot flushes to the head especially during abdominal pain.
Bad breath in the morning.

Mentals & Generals
Anxiety attacks.
Insomnia.
Mood swings.
Fear of heights.

Family History
Mother: allergic to bee stings and penicillin.
Father's mother: breast cancer, stomach cancer

Medication
Mintec (antispasmodic for IBS pain)

Investigations

Coeliac test (gliadin antibodies) is negative.

Prescription 1

Cina 200: One dose every second day in reducing doses over a three month period. I chose *Cina* because:

- History of gastroenteritis
- Teeth grinding
- Irritability, restlessness and anxiety
- Recurring diarrhoea with coeliac disease ruled out
- Migraines, insomnia, anxiety oversensitivity of the nervous system)
- Salicylate food sensitivity.

I suspected this was a case of post-gastroenteritis parasitosis.

***Follow up**: Three months later*

I saw Ann once per month for three months. After aggravation of symptoms in the first week, the monthly follow up consultations showed a steady improvement: fatty foods did not trigger symptoms; the sleep, teeth grinding and also the anxiety ameliorated; the frequency and severity of the cramping and diarrhoea symptoms improved. The migraine headaches persisted but were less frequent. The frequent colds improved.

Prescription 2

Sycotic Co 200: One dose, then as needed to hold. I chose *Sycotic Co* because three months treatment with *Cina* had significantly ameliorated but not resolved the symptoms. The extreme episodes of diarrhoea with pain suggested chronic inflammation of the gastrointestinal tract. She was also irritable, both keynotes for this Bowel nosode.

***Follow up**: Seven weeks later*

Ann had 13 bouts of diarrhoea with abdominal pain, waking at night regardless of food (over the summer holidays). The teeth grinding recommenced. However the migraine headaches and tiredness were somewhat better and she was still free of anxiety. I felt the case was not moving forward, so I returned to *Cina* and also gave a specific medicine for the diarrhoea and griping pain.

Prescription 3

Cina 200 and *Mercurius cor 30* alternating every second day for a month; then *Cina 200* every other day; *Mercurius cor 30* as needed for a month. She was advised to follow a low salicylate diet. After one month reduce *Cina 200* to every third day, then every fourth day, then as needed, over three months. Re-introduce salicylates gradually. *Cina* remained an essential medicine for the patient, since withdrawal resulted in relapse. It was clear that another medicine was needed to resolve symptoms, so I selected *Mercurius cor* purely on the particular symptoms. Further amelioration was achieved, but low grade symptoms persisted. *Lycopodium 30* was also used at a later time, with some good but partial relief of symptoms. Still the patient was not moving to cure even though her symptoms were well managed by *Cina* and the other medicines.

Follow up: *Three months later*

Although the patient remained vastly improved, *Cina* needed frequent repetition to sustain it. Thus I chose a new medicine to move the case further. As described in Chapter 3, when a patient responds well to *Cina* but relapses, *Trichinose Nosode* is well indicated.

Trichinose Nosode 30: One dose every second day.

Follow up: *Two months later*

There was an aggravation ('gastro bug') five weeks after commencing *Trichinose Nosode*, with vomiting, diarrhoea and bloating. Since that time she has been completely symptom free. Since then she has taken no homeopathic medicine, and *remains free of insomnia, anxiety, migraines and abdominal pain and diarrhoea*. The patient is able to tolerate salicylates without incident.

Ann was discharged symptom free.

Discussion

- I considered this was a case of post-gastroenteritis parasitosis.

- *Mercurius cor* and *Lycopodium* afforded symptomatic relief, but did not appear to play a significant role in the ultimate removal of symptoms.

- Note the aggravation from *Trichinose Nosode* five weeks after it was commenced. Aggravations this far into the treatment are not always expected, yet since the patient has remained symptom free since that time, it is certain that her 'gastro bug' was an aggravation.

- A more direct path of cure for this patient might have been a course of *Cina* followed by *Trichinose Nosode,* as described in the treatment protocols for intestinal parasites. Certainly, while she was taking *Cina* she remained vastly improved, but not cured, in all her symptoms. *Trichinose Nosode* is discussed at p 55.

Case 2: Iatrogenic cause of IBS

This case illustrates how IBS may be caused by allopathic medication, and how repeated use of a homeopathic medicine may be useful. In this case the allopathic and homeopathic medicine exert their respective influences simultaneously.

Jack, Male, 56, presented with these symptoms:

Irritable bowel syndrome for three years: intermittent explosive and episodic diarrhoea, with abdominal cramps and flatulence occurring before bowel movements, lasting up to two weeks per episode. This followed after a kidney transplant two and a half years previously. He is taking immuno-suppressive medication to prevent donor organ rejection. I suspect the allopathic medication is the cause of his IBS. His diarrhoea is accompanied by fatigue, weakness and poor sleep. Understandably, he is anxious about his health and exhausted by his frequent diarrhoea. He presents as withdrawn and avoiding being the centre of attention.

History
Asthma until age 20.
Glandular fever.
Kidney failure & transplant.
Urethral leakage.
Gout.
Osteoporosis.
Hip replacement.
Peritonitis.
Rectal itch.

Particulars
Vision: floaters.
Glue ear.

Mentals & Generals
"Fear of the future always holds me back."
"Always seeking freedom in whatever way I can."
Allergy to dust, pollens and cats.

Family History
Father: bladder cancer.
Father's family: skin cancer.
Mother's family: polycystic kidney disease.

Medications
Tacrolimas (Immunomodifier)
CellCept (Immunomodifier)
Prednisolone (anti-inflammatory)
Cardizem (antihypertensive)
Avrapro (antihypertensive)
Progout (antihyperuricaemic)
Fosamax (mineral treatment for osteoporosis)
Ferro-gradumet (iron supplement)
Calcitriol (calcium supplement)

Prescription 1
Cina 200: One dose every second day. With the history of rectal itch, I wanted to exclude the possibility of parasitosis.

Follow up: *One month later*
The diarrhoea symptoms aggravated for four days, improved for two weeks, and then relapsed. The abdominal cramps improved. The sleep improved slightly. From this response I considered that parasites were not the cause of this man's IBS, despite the history of rectal itching. I felt certain his symptoms were iatrogenic. One or more of his allopathic medications, which were nonetheless essential for his survival, was probably producing the IBS symptoms.

Prescription 2
Morgan Bach 200: Take as needed at onset of diarrhoea episodes for two months.

Follow up: *Three months later*
With each required dose of *Morgan Bach 200* (every few weeks) the patient's diarrhoea stopped immediately and the patient lasted for two to three weeks without any diarrhoea, followed by some minor episodes. After two months the diarrhoea and abdominal pain returned. (The patient however had been taking antibiotics for his flu,

which may have prevented the medicine working further.) *Morgan Bach 1M* was then tried without further improvement. I therefore considered the effect of this Bowel nosode had been extinguished. The patient described his diarrhoea episodes as having an insecure feeling over his bowel motions. He could not tell if he were going to pass flatulence or diarrhoea. This meant he could not go out when he was in his diarrhoea cycle. This 'insecurity of the rectum', resulting in faecal incontinence, is described in the treatment section at p 86. It is a specific symptom in *Aloe.*

Prescription 3
Aloe 200: One dose as needed, whenever the diarrhoea occurs.

Follow up: *Six months later*
Jack reported he was "the best I've been in years" using *Aloe 200* as needed. This good response to the medicine continued over the next six months. Over this time I also treated him for a chest infection with wheezing; gastric reflux; and urinary problems related to benign prostate enlargement.

Discussion

- The patient's IBS was caused by his essential allopathic medication necessary to prevent rejection of his transplanted kidney.

- *Aloe 200* managed his IBS symptoms with confidence, without interfering with the action of his allopathic medication.

- *Cina* did not hold, and in hindsight was an inappropriate prescription, given the patient's history and causation.

- *Morgan Bach* was used based on the patient's mentals (introversion and avoiding company) with some success.

Case 3: A Puzzling Case

This unusual case illustrates that pathological prescribing is sometimes the only way to find a cure for the patient. The need for careful patient examination, knowledge of symptomatology and diagnosis and *Materia Medica* are highlighted here.

Sara, Female, 8, presented with these symptoms:

'Chest pains and ear aches', for the past two years. Periodically, usually twice weekly, she would complain of suddenly feeling very cold. She would then experience increasingly severe sharp, stabbing and continuous chest pain, which could last for several hours. The pain came on gradually, often after dinner, and sometimes after exertion, and would then increase slowly until it became unbearable. At these times she would just want to be still and keep warm. In more than half of the episodes, she experienced sharp pain in the ears (a concomitant symptom.) Sara was afebrile during attacks. Analgesics had little effect. Antacid medications also had no effect. The only way for her to find slight relief was to have a hot bath. On the several occasions when Sara was taken to Accident and Emergency, medical staff did not believe she was in pain because all her medical investigations had been normal. Investigations were:

- Barium swallow
- Cardiac assessment
- A range of blood tests: all normal.

After a number of hospital visits and investigations, the parents were told Sara had 'irritable bowel syndrome'.

On Examination

Middle ear was normal.

When asked to touch the spot where she felt the pain she pointed to the right of and just below the sternum, in the epigastrium (ie not the chest as was related by the patient).

Mentals & Generals

- A cold child, 'always cold'.
- A 'bubbly, bouncy child, who is sometimes moody at home'.

- She 'handles her sickness well' (thus inviting disbelief from her doctors).
- Fears: cockroaches.
- Stubborn 'when things don't go her way'.
- Food aversions: 'anything different'.

Medical history

Birth: Acrocyanosis, which spontaneously resolved.
Two years: Croup followed by bronchitis.
No other events until the current symptoms.

Family history

Father: gastric reflux and ulcer.
Mother: food sensitivities, allergy to dye, fibroids, nasal polyps.
No other significant history.

Onset

Sara caught a cold, after which a persistent cough developed which did not resolve. *Seretide* gradually reduced the cough. *When the cough resolved, her current symptoms began.*

Discussion

Too often these patients are passed off as 'hypochondriacal' because they defy diagnosis. Yet there was no evidence to me that this was the case. The mother, an accountant, was very ordered and down to earth and the child was entirely consistent in her rendering of the symptoms (although understandably, she confused chest with upper right epigastrium).

I began by asking her to show me where her pain was. She pointed to her epigastrium, just below and to the right of her sternum. Such an instance illuminates the importance of physical examination.

I thought about all the different ailments which could produce Sara's symptoms. Considering the character, cyclic nature and location of the pains, I decided the only logical cause was cholecystitis, even though this is rare in children. Biliary calculi would be most unlikely in such a young patient. My tentative diagnosis was therefore non-calculi cholecystitis or 'gallbladder colic'.

Prescription 1
Carduus mar 30: One dose every second day (and every 20 minutes when the pain occurs). *Carduus mar* was chosen because it addresses epigastric pain caused by cholecystitis occurring periodically. There is no pain between attacks. Making a clear diagnosis enabled me to narrow medicine selection to a small number of gallbladder medicines. [27]

Follow up: *Six weeks later*
Sara improved steadily on this medicine, which was repeated every second day for six weeks. Her ear pain resolved completely within the first week of treatment. By week six her symptoms had plateaued, with no further improvement.

I thought more about the common, and less common, causes of cholecystitis, with particular reference to children. Cholecystitis is usually caused by occlusion of the common bile duct. A rare cause of cholecystitis is occlusion of the bile duct due to ascarides.[28] Could intestinal parasites be the cause of the duct occlusion? *Carduus mar* had greatly improved the case, but the improvement had stalled.

Prescription 2
Cina 200: One dose every second day. *Carduus mar* to be used only if attacks occur.

Third Visit: *10 weeks later*
After a further 10 weeks all the symptoms were gone and *the original cough which preceded the pain attacks had returned.* I had previously told the mother that the cough might come back, and that this should be seen as a good sign, with complete cure possible. So she understood not to medicate the cough with *Seretide* or other allopathic medication, as she had done earlier. We cannot understand completely how the allopathic treatment suppressed the symptoms of the disease in this case, but with the reappearance of the cough we were observing an outstanding example of Hering's Law.

---

[27] The treatment of gallbladder disease is detailed in *Mastering Homeopathy: Accurate Daily Prescribing for a Successful Practice,* ibid.
[28] *Merck Manual*, 17th ed, p 1260

Her cough began with high fever and chills +++ worse at 3 to 4 am. 'She is always a chilly child.'
There was yellow to brown chest phlegm with no chest pain and she had a headache with the cough.

The cough had appeared briefly one month before, *when the epigastric symptoms disappeared; the epigastric symptoms then reappeared once the cough cleared.* Now the same obstinate cough, which had occurred two years prior, before the start of her 'chest pain', had re-established.

This was the next crucial part of the treatment, since the correct medicine would address the underlying respiratory susceptibility without suppressing the symptoms again.

Prescription 3
Silicea 200: Two doses.

I chose *Silicea* because:

- Very chilly patient (with history of acrocyanosis)
- History of obstinate cough
- Susceptibility to respiratory illness evident with bronchitis at age two
- Stubborn in nature.

Follow up: *Four weeks later*
The fevers, cough and chest symptoms cleared within a few days of taking *Silicea* and this little girl has returned to her normal life.

Discussion

- If I had repertorised the case I do not think I would have found the correct medicine.

- It was essential to fully understand the origin of her presenting symptoms in order to prescribe.

- Knowledge of *Materia Medica* to match the presenting pathology was essential to find the correct medicine. The notion that homeopaths can prescribe on symptomatology alone works in some cases, but in others, medicine selection is entirely dependent on an accurate assessment of the physiology of the symptoms.

- The original symptoms, suppressed by allopathic medicine, returned, according to Hering's Law. Similarly, her presenting symptoms abated while a deeper layer of disease suppression (the original cough) temporarily returned.

- Her constitutional medicine (*Silicea)* was required once the original symptoms resurfaced.

- At a follow up visit one year later, the patient remained symptom free for most of that year, with two small, 'inconsequential' episodes in the last month of the old pain. On both occasions Sara had been exposed to cold air, and a slight pain had manifested for about 30 seconds afterwards.. One year to the day after giving *Silicea,* I repeated the dose. The patient has had no further pain since that time, nor has she had any colds.

Case 4: Parasitosis in a Child

Most cases of unknown abdominal pain in children result from parasitosis.

Phillip, Male, 5, presented with these symptoms:

Diarrhoea with abdominal pain since he was a baby, with flatulence and smelly stools, and more recently with daily vomiting. His main complaint was ongoing abdominal pain.

History
Prolonged cough.
Ear infections.
Snoring.
Adenoidectomy at age four.
Bilateral grommets at age four.
Sleep walking.

Particulars
Spoon-shaped nails (can be a sign of chronic respiratory illness).
Perspiration: head, soles of feet.
Flushed appearance.
Huge appetite.

Mentals
Placid but irritable when ill.
Stubborn.

Family History
Mother as a child: eczema, bronchitis.
Mother as an adult: eczema, allergies to medication.
Father as an adult: eczema.

***Prescription* 1**
Nux vom 30 and *Stannum met* 200: One dose on alternate days.

Follow up: *Five weeks later*

The child's stools became formed for the first time in his life. His bowels were moving easier twice a day; the flatulence was better; his appetite was less ravenous.

Continue *Nux vom 30* and *Stannum met 200* : One dose every third day, alternating.

Follow up: *One month later*
The child now had a healthy appetite. He had not suffered any diarrhoea. He had abdominal pain only once "after eating too much", he said. The flushing had improved and he was perspiring rather more.

Continue *Nux vom 30 and Stannum met 200*: One dose of each per month for six months. The patient was then discharged, symptom free.

Discussion

- The chief complaint was ongoing abdominal pain, with diarrhoea, and ear, nose and throat (ENT) symptoms. There was no rectal itch. Thus *Nux and Stannum* were chosen in preference to *Cina,* as described in the treatment protocol at p 53.

- Had the patient not improved on homeopathic medicine, referral for Coeliac disease assessment would have been recommended.

Case 5: Parasitosis & Gallbladder

This case illustrates a dual treatment protocol using homeopathic medicine plus herbal tinctures as Boericke used to bring rapid relief to the patient.

Sue, Female, 35, presented with the following symptoms which had occurred intermittently for some years, but were worse after travel in the developing world four months earlier.

Abdominal bloating and griping pain.
Explosive diarrhoea.
Flatulence.
Sensation of blockage in the epigastrium.
Reflux after garlic and spicy foods.
Aggravation: fatty foods+++, dairy foods, bread.
Allergy to: shellfish, *Ibobrufen*.

The above symptoms had occurred intermittently for some years, but were worse after travel in the developing world four months previously.

History
Chronic cystitis.
A bout of depression for one year at age 34.

Particulars
Itching flaking scalp, can scratching until it bleeds.
Polycystic ovary syndrome with infertility.

Mentals
Impatient and irritable.
Unmotivated.
Lethargic.
Restless sleep.

Family History
Mother: migraines.
Father: rheumatic fever and valvular disease.
Other: asthma, adult onset diabetes.

Prescription 1

Cina 200: One dose every second day; *Chelidonium tincture*: 15 drops twice daily.

Follow up: *One month later*

The diarrhoea and abdominal pain improved after three days, plateaued, then completely resolved after ten days. The aggravation from fatty foods also cleared. The patients restless sleep was much improved.

Sue followed up with medicines for the psoriasis of the scalp.

Discussion

- The recent history of overseas travel aggravating her IBS suggested intestinal parasites.

- The patient's griping pain was caused by flatulence as a result of her food sensitivities and inability to tolerate *fatty* foods, the latter suggestive of gallbladder stasis. Accordingly, *Chelidonium tincture* was given in addition to *Cina*, with complete and rapid resolution of symptoms.

- Food sensitivities usually improve when gastro-intestinal treatment resolves the complaint.

- Once again I noticed a relationship between parasitosis and disturbed sleep, both of which improved after *Cina.*

Case 6: 'Never Well Since' and Post-viral Syndrome

This unusual case illustrates the sometimes long process to identify the curative medicine. Whilst revealing the therapeutic potential of several medicines, only one could produce a cure.

Christine, Female, 30, presented with these symptoms:

Chronic diarrhoea with abdominal pain over the previous three years. The episodes of diarrhoea are severe, lasting from two days to four weeks. The patient is a neat, intelligent woman with a good sense of humour. Her debilitating IBS has not impacted on her emotional state at all.

History
Migraine headaches at 13 years.

Particulars
Sudden nausea of a few days duration unrelated to the diarrhoea.
Headaches with dull pain behind the eyes, occurring every second day.

Migraines with fast onset, with partial vision loss from the left eye, with vomiting, and worse for change in the weather, more frequent and severe with age.

Facial eczema: itchy eyelids.

Generals
Energy levels rated five out of 10.
Generally feels unwell most of the time.

Family History
Mother: osteoporosis.
Father: migraines.
Father's mother: cancer of the lung.
Father's father: cancer, vascular complaints.

Medications
Oral contraceptive pill.

Investigations
Colonoscopy and gastroscopy normal. (No coeliac disease.)

Prescription 1
Mercurius cor 30 : One dose every second day. I chose this medicine entirely on the presenting particulars of abdominal gripe with diarrhoea.

Follow up: *Three weeks later*
The patient had a good improvement with just one bout of diarrhoea. Fatigue slightly better.

Prescription 2
Mercurius cor 30 and Entamoeba histolytica 30: One dose on alternate days, with advice to avoid wheat and preservatives in the diet. I tried to enhance the action of the medicine by alternating with an intestinal pathogen in potency. This was an experiment which produced no clear result.

Follow up: *Three weeks later*
The diarrhoea and abdominal pain symptoms relapsed while she was on holidays. She now adds these new symptoms:
Skin is sensitive to perfumes and to alcohol.
'Restless legs' at night.
Headaches improved while avoiding wheat and preservatives.

***Prescription* 3**
Morgan Pure 30: One dose every second day. Use *Mercurius cor 30* as needed. *Mercurius cor* was an effective medicine, but it was not moving the patient to cure. Thus I prescribed a Bowel nosode. I chose a *Morgan* because of the bilious and nauseas factor in her symptoms.

Follow up: *Four weeks later*
The diarrhoea, headaches, eczema, sleep and "restless legs" all improved.

***Prescription* 4**
Morgan Pure 30: One dose every second day, with advice to try re-introducing yeast in the diet.

Follow up: *Five weeks later*
The improvement in the diarrhoea and other symptoms held, however the patient was still intolerant to yeast.

***Prescription* 5**
Nux vom 30 and Stannum met 200: One dose on alternate days. I wanted to see if there was a parasitic factor in her IBS.

Follow up: *Two months later*
The patient stopped taking the *Nux vom 30 and Stannum 200* as the diarrhoea and nausea returned after two weeks. However after that she felt substantially better with just one bout of diarrhoea. Although she was sleeping well, she would wake *unrefreshed* (new symptom). In terms of her energy and wellbeing, she felt *worse*. Since her generals were worse, the prescription was incorrect. Thus I return to safe ground.

Prescription 6
Merc cor 30 alternating with *Morgan Pure 30* every other day.

Follow up: *Two months later*
Mostly well, with no diarrhoea at all, but occasional abdominal cramps. She uses *Mercurius cor* when this occurs which, after several doses, relieves the cramps. However, generally her nausea and tiredness persist, with her energy levels remaining only five out of 10.

She then relates this information, not previously disclosed: her symptoms started after her then partner contracted Infectious Mononucleosis (Glandular Fever). He then went on to develop Chronic Fatigue Syndrome. She did not develop concurrent viral symptoms but *this was the start point for her presenting symptoms.*

Prescription 7
Coxsackievirus 30: One dose every second day.

Follow up: *Six weeks later*
Symptom free: including complete resolution of fatigue, sleep problem, restless legs and abdominal pain. She experienced some

aggravation from the medicine: a sore throat, which occurred each day after she took the medicine. (I instruct her to continue taking the *Coxsackievirus* once weekly until she no longer experiences any aggravation from it, after which time she can challenge wheat and yeast.)

Follow up: *Two months later*
She remains symptom-free, despite wheat and yeast being back on her menu. No further medicine is needed and she is discharged.

Discussion

- *Mercurius cor* was a specific treatment for her symptom particulars, but it did not advance her to cure.

- *Morgan Pure* improved her general and specific symptoms, but it also failed to advance her to cure.

- *Nux vom and Stannum met* possibly aggravated the case. Because this was not a case parasitosis, these medicines were ineffective or inappropriate prescriptions. In hindsight, a parasitic-induced IBS causing severe diarrhoea would be likely to provoke some kind of emotional disturbance too, as we have seen in other cases. There appeared to be no emotional disturbance in this case.

- *Coxsackievirus* was the most correct medicine because it is specific for 'never well since Glandular Fever', see pp 69 and 77. Even though Christine did not contract Glandular Fever, her exposure to it through her partner initiated a disease process. It is unclear how this happens, but it has been well noted, particularly in the early days of Chronic Fatigue Syndrome, that carers could sometimes develop the same symptoms as their patients.

Case 7: Constipation

Treating patients who take many allopathic medications can be confusing. This is one such case, with long-standing constipation and systemic symptoms.

Ilma, Female, 54, presented with these symptoms:
Life-long constipation, with ineffectual urging. Bowel motions sometimes only once every seven days.

History

Undiagnosed transient ailment in her 20s where she was unable to walk unassisted after birth of second child.
In her 30s, child born stillborn.
In her 40s, seizures during sleep (undiagnosed).

Particulars

Burning pain in legs worse for walking.
Headaches.
High blood pressure

Mentals & Generals

Fastidious.
Fear of the dark.
Dizzy spells once or twice a month.

Medications

Lamictal (anticonvulsant)
Natrilix (antihypertensive)
Tenormin (beta-adrenergic blocker)
Pravachol (hypolipidaemic)
Progout (hyperuricaemic)
Aspirin (anticoagulant)

Prescription 1

Bryonia 200: One dose every second day. *Bryonia* is a specific for chronic, dry, hard constipation with headache. It is the most frequent medicine I use for chronic constipation in adults.

***Follow up**: Three weeks later*
The patient had bowel motions most days, but still with ineffectual urging'. She was mostly free of headaches. The dizziness remained the same.

Continue *Bryonia 200:* One dose every second day.

Follow up: Four weeks later
The bowels were moving easier, and mostly every day. Her headaches and dizziness had improved, she was sleeping well and the burning pain in the legs was improved.

Continue *Bryonia 200:* One dose every second day.

***Follow up:** Four weeks later*
Constipation and urging are now gone, with bowel motions every day. The headaches and dizziness are now gone. The burning in legs is mostly gone.

Continue *Bryonia 200:* One dose every third day. The treatment plan is: slowly reduce frequency of dose, by one day per month until the medicine is no longer needed.

Discussion

- This patient is very dependent on allopathic medication. Her symptoms all improve on a homeopathic medicine prescribed on her particulars of long-standing dry constipation with headaches. Her dizziness and leg symptoms are referred from her bowel problem, since they too improve on *Bryonia*.
- One side effect is that *Pravachol,* causes her to feel bloated. In patients who are heavily medicated it is sometimes difficult to know which are natural symptoms and which are drug-induced.
- Treatment plan: continue *Bryonia* in doses of decreasing frequency. If the patient wishes to revise her allopathic treatment regime at some time (which she does not wish to do now), her homeopathic treatment plan can be revised. Until then it is not possible to go deeper into the case or to treat constitutionally.

Case 8: Anxiety-related IBS

I explored a number of causes in this case, because as a general rule of thumb, when the patient has localised abdominal pain, there is likely to be a cause other than anxiety.

Jamie, Female, 43, presented with these symptoms:

Abdominal pain on the *left* side, since cholecystectomy, two years prior.
Diarrhoea when stressed.
Difficulty sleeping.
This patient presented as a timid woman who did not stand up well to her verbally aggressive husband. I suspected this was part of her IBS problem.

History
Tonsillectomy at age five.
Appendicectomy at age eight.
Lumpectomy (left breast) in her 20s.
Removal of gall bladder in her 30s.

Particulars
Abdominal pain in the left iliac fossa with back pain worse after eating, better for passing wind.
Belching.
Phlegm and tickle in the throat.

Mentals & Generals
Low energy levels.
Some sleep disturbance.
Dreams of protecting children but failing.

Family History
Mother: heart disease, high blood pressure.
Father: prostate cancer.

Prescription 1
Trichinose Nosode 30 and *Lycopodium 30*: One dose on alternate days. Essentially, I chose *Lycopodium* because:

- It rarely fails in reducing flatulent abdominal bloating
- Although a clearly intelligent woman, Jamie became confused when 'put on the spot'.

I was not sure if there was also a parasitic component, so I alternated *Lycopodium* with the *Trichinose Nosode.*

***Follow up**: Four weeks later*
The patient was free of diarrhoea. There was an immediate improvement in the bloating and abdominal pain – as well as improvements in the throat tickle, belching, back pain and in sleeping. She still has some anxiety and confusion when making decisions.

Continue *Trichinose Nosode 30* and *Lycopodium 30:* One dose on alternate days.

***Follow up:** Four weeks later*
All the physical complaints improved required no further treatment. Her anxiety and sleep quality were greatly improved.

I decide to target her emotional state when she reveals that her husband is impossible to please. He loses his temper and then she feels reprimanded, intimidated and humiliated in front of people. She wants acceptance from her husband and validation that she is capable. [Her husband has just started receiving *Lycopodium* with some improvement in his temper noted].

Prescription 2
Staphysagria 1M: One dose.

***Follow up:** Four weeks later*
Jamie is feeling well. Anxiety and sleep difficulty are much better. No IBS symptoms.

Discussion

- There was a significant anxiety pattern without the symptoms suggestive of *Cina.* I decided to try *Trichinose Nosode,* to cover any parasitic cause of her illness. I am not sure if this medicine was needed.

- *Lycopodium* was also prescribed because of her lack of self confidence, and because it would reduce her abdominal bloating, affording her immediate symptomatic relief. Her anxiety and poor sleep patterns improved commensurate with her bowel symptoms.

- *Staphysagria* was then given for her mental symptoms ('ailments from reprimand and humiliation'). It was also indicated for the possible aetiology: 'Never well since abdominal surgery', in this case her gallbladder surgery. After this medicine, her anxiety and sleep were much better and her bowel symptoms were absent.

Case 9: Post-enteritis Parasitosis

The full array of chronic parasitosis symptoms are displayed in this case.

Peter, Male, 24, presented with these symptoms:

Skin problems: dandruff, warts, tinea, moles.
Food sensitivities: with gluten, alcohol, spices, meaty, dairy, lemon, overeating.
Gastric reflux with obstinate helicobacter pylori unresponsive to antibiotics.
Chronic diarrhoea with occasional blood smear < dairy, chicken, overseas travel.
Morning nausea, fatigue and lethargy
Post nasal drip and ongoing sinus.
Occasional insomnia.
Occasional rectal itch < after alcohol.
Abdominal bloating.
Weight loss.

The patient was an aloof young man who tended to be irritable at home. He had travelled extensively in the developing world and contracted traveller's diarrhoea there, which had at times been bloody. This is a common presentation of post-enteritis parasitosis.

History
Recurring bronchitis, not currently active.
Asthma as a child.
Multiple courses of antibiotics and antifungal creams.
His worst episode of diarrhoea was in South America where he was very ill for some weeks and lost much weight.
Teeth grinding.
Moderate marijuana use.

Mentals
Irritable.
Presents as aloof.
Some insomnia with anxiety.

Prescription 1

Cina 200: One dose every second day.
Chelidonium tincture: 15 drops in water three times daily before food. While not essential, I prescribe *Chelidonium* in addition to *Cina* to hasten an improvement in his food sensitivities. Morning nausea, fatigue and intolerance to spices, meat and chicken suggest sluggish bile function.

Follow up: *Five weeks later*
All symptoms resolved on *Cina,* including a vast improvement is his food sensitivities. Consequently I maintained the same medicine at decreasing frequency until symptom-free. I also ask him to monitor his stool for any further presence of blood or mucus, with advice to seek a colonoscopy if these symptoms return.

Discussion
This is a clear case of intestinal parasitosis given these typical symptoms:

- Diarrhoea aggravated during travel in South America
- Weight loss
- Teeth grinding
- Irritability
- Insomnia
- Rectal itch
- Food sensitivities +++
- Fatigue, nausea, lethargy.

This young man had not been referred for a colonoscopy, despite his history of haemorrhagic diarrhoea. This is certainly a red bullet symptom for a serious pathology. However, his presenting symptoms and history suggest that he has a chronic parasitic infection. I commence homeopathic treatment and strongly urge a colonoscopy if there is no improvement by the time of his five-week follow up. While one thinks of *Mercurius sol* for haemorrhagic diarrhoea, his symptoms are very strong for *Cina. Mercurius* would be appropriate for him if he were in an acute phase of diarrhoea. However, his disease is chronic, and very serious.

Follow up: *Five weeks later*
All his symptoms improve rapidly on *Cina.* Peter's only complaint was his continuing food sensitivity: some slight nausea, fatigue and occasional loose stool after eating the offending foods. His diarrhoea was much better. His energy had improved.

Plan
Continue *Cina* until all symptoms are resolved. As the patient did not keep his follow-up the outcome is not known.

Case 10: Chronic Sinusitis with IBS

Jill, Female, 29, presented with these symptoms:
Urgent bowel movements with abdominal pain for the past nine years.
Fatigue < mornings.

History
Glandular fever at age 16.
Nose fracture.
Adverse reaction to antibiotics.

Particulars
Pale stool.
Sinusitis with blocked nose, post nasal drip with thick green mucus and blocked nose.

Mentals
Fear in a crowd.

Family History
Heart disease.
Grandmother: breast cancer.
Grandfather: nasal cancer.
Stomach ulcer.
Thyroid condition.

Prescription 1
Teucrium 200: One dose every second day.

Follow up: *Four weeks later*
The abdominal pain was 100% improved; the stool was darker. The general sinus symptoms were somewhat improved. The patient was sleeping better. She also said her skin and headaches, two things not mentioned before, were better.

Continue *Teucrium 200*: One dose every third day for four weeks.

Follow up: *Four weeks later*
The patient relapsed, experiencing increased upset stomach and flatulence. She noticed further aggravation after eating fatty food:

especially worse in the morning. However, the patient graded her symptoms as 70 per cent better since before commencing treatment. I queried her again about the onset of her IBS nine years ago. On reflecting she said it was after she had started the oral contraceptive pill. Yet since she had discontinued this 12 months ago she did not feel it was relevant.

Prescription 2
Folliculinum 30: One dose every second day until next visit. As described, this medicine is specific for never well since the use of synthetic oestrogens.

Follow up: *Two weeks later*
There was immediate improvement in bowel symptoms. She rated her symptoms as 70 per cent better since starting homeopathic treatment.

***Prescription 3*:**
Trichinose Nosode 30: One dose every second day.

Follow up: *Eight weeks later*
The patient had very occasional urgent bowel motions. Both the sinus symptoms and the blocked nose were substantially improved. Fatigue was better.

Prescription 4
Teucrium 200: One dose every second day, plus *Trichinose Nosode 30*: One dose every third day. Continue until all symptoms are resolved.

Discussion

- Since the patient had a combination of IBS (diarrhoea) and sinus symptoms, with post nasal discharge and chronic blockage, with the possibility of nasal polyps, I chose *Teucrium* to cover the sinus and any possible parastic component. When improvement stalled, I added *Trichinose Nosode*. I decided to try a combination treatment at the end, which was effective in resolving symptoms.
- However, an obstacle to cure was her past use of the oral contraceptive pill. I have found that even if used many years

prior to the consultation, it can have lasting effects on sinus, gut and genito-urinary symptoms. *Folliculinum* is specific for removing the effects of synthetic oestrogens.

- The history of glandular fever did not appear to be responsible for symptoms.

Case 11: Emotional and Behavioural IBS

This case illustrates a case of paediatric IBS *not* caused by intestinal parasites.

Billy, Male, 11, presents with these symptoms:

Constipation with lack of sphincter control. Still not properly toilet trained he would experience faecal incontinence once a week. The stool was painful with hard pellets and he was scared of toilets. He had flatulence and belching. He craved sweet food. At school he had poor concentration. He could not sit still, disturbing the class by pushing and hitting. He did not have friends. 'Nobody likes me'. He responded well to, and desired, affection from his mother. He was stubborn and would have tantrums 'destroying a room'. Afterwards he would stare into space. He had an anxiety about germs, regularly wiping his drink bottle. At twelve months of age he had asthma and eczema. Two of his aunts suffered from irritable bowel syndrome.

History
One year of age: restless sleep waking every two hours.
Asthma, eczema.
Age four: ear infections, grommets, adenoidectomy.

Particulars
Stool: hard pellets.
Bowel very blocked preventing regular daily stool.
Flatulence, belching.
Desire for sweets.

Mentals & Generals
Poor concentration at school; very stubborn; lots of aggressive tantrums.
Wants all the attention.
Fear of going to the toilet.
Anxiety about germs.
Desires sugar+++ and aggravates from it.
Restlessness.
Restless sleep.

Family History
Grandfather: asthma.
Mother: post-natal depression.
Two aunts: Irritable Bowel Syndrome.
Sister: anxiety.

Medications
Benefiber (laxative)
Movicol (laxative)

Prescription 1
Saccharum 200: One dose every second day for 10 days.

Follow up: *Two weeks later*
No faecal incontinence; less flatulence; improved sleep; calmer behaviour.

Continue *Saccharum 200*: One dose every third day with advice to avoid wheat, sugar and foods with preservatives and colourings.

Follow up: Three weeks later
No faecal incontinence; no flatulence; better concentration and behaviour.

Continue *Saccharum 200*: One dose every fourth day.

Follow up: *Four weeks later*
The child had had two small bowel accidents. His symptoms, particularly his behaviour, relapsed when he had chocolate or preservatives in the diet.

Continue *Saccharum 200*: One dose every fourth day.

Follow up: *Three weeks later*
Generally improved, however the child occasionally passed liquid stool after eating wheat.

Continue *Saccharum 200*: One dose once a week. Avoid wheat, sugar, food colourings and preservatives.

Follow up: *Four weeks later*
Still generally improved, however the child would be aggressive, stubborn and irritable after eating sugar, chocolate and food colouring.

Continue *Saccharum 200*: One dose once per week.

Follow up: Five weeks later
The child was doing well at school. His behaviour was better depending on his diet, he could tolerate some wheat. He still faecally incontinent on occasions. I felt *Saccharum* had achieved all it was going to so I chose a new prescription.

Prescription2
Lycopodium 200: One dose every third day with advice to continue dietary restrictions.

Follow up
The patient continued to improve on *Lycopodium* with further improvement in food aggravations, and considerably less incidence ot soiling.

Discussion

- *Saccharum* was chosen because of the aggressive, restless behaviour, aggravation from sugar, poor concentration and desire for constant attention.

- *Lycopodium* was chosen to further improve the case, after *Saccharum* seemed to have run its course. With *Lycopodium* the food tolerance improved further, and the patient was better in terms of concentration, tantrums, soiling, provided food additives were restricted.

- A useful profile of the *Saccharum* child can be found in Tinus Smits' article in *Homoeopathic Links*, Volume 8, Autumn 1995 3/95 pp 28-36.

Case 12: A Complex, Multi-Layered Case

Felicity, Female, 29, presents with these symptoms:

She has suffered most of her life with diarrhoea, constipation, abdominal pain, which have led to many hospitalisations. She is a professional, career-oriented single woman. My impression is that she is guarded, drives herself hard, is successful but unfulfilled.

History
Viral meningitis age six.
Severe abdominal pain with recurring bowel obstruction between 12-17 years of age.
Ovarian tumor removed.
Appendicectomy.
Lapband surgery for gastric reflux.
Sphincterotomy.
Surgery for endometriosis.
Duodenal and peptic ulcer.
Several bouts of gastroenteritis (salmonella poisoning).
Yersinia enterocolitica infection.
Long term use of antibiotics for chlamydia, salmonella, yersinia enterocolitica.
Allergy to cats.

Particulars
Shifting abdominal pain in lower part of abdomen not relieved by bowel movements (ie classical IBS symptom).
Severe bloating.
Itchy nose and throat.

Mentals & Generals
Fatigue.
High achiever, competitive.

Family History
Father: hypertension, elevated cholesterol; pituitary tumor.

Medications
Depo-provera (gonadal hormone)

Prescription 1

Lycopodium 30 and *Cina 200*: One dose on alternate days. With such a long history of bowel infections I consider she has post-infective IBS, and prescribe *Cina.* I add *Lycopodium* to give her immediate relief from the severe bloating.

Follow up: *Four weeks later*

The patient reported she felt considerably better after ten days, then had a slight relapse. She was *free of diarrhoea but not constipation.* She reported straining and incomplete evacuation. The itchy throat, nose and rectum had mostly resolved. She had one day of depression – a recurring problem – but generally was not as tired.

Prescription 2

Nux vom 30 and *Stannum met 200*: One dose on alternate days. As her symptoms had changed to *constipation-dominant* IBS, thus it was appropriate to amend the prescription choice. Avoid salicylates in the diet.

Follow up: *Four weeks later*

All symptoms improved including better stress management. The constipation was slightly better, achieving complete evacuation.

Continue *Nux vom 30* and *Stannum met 200*: One dose of each every third day with advice to continue avoiding salicylates in the diet.

Follow up: *Four weeks later*

Improvement maintained. Food with salicylates continued to aggravate, causing bloating, throat and nose itch, eczema.

Prescription 3

Morgan-Gaertner 30 and *Morgan Bach 30 (mixed):* One dose daily for three days, then once a week. Continue *Nux vom 30* and *Stannum met 200*: One dose alternating every third day. The intercurrent use of these Bowel nosodes was to revitalise the action of the medicines.

The *Morgans* were chosen because of the patient's depression and congestion, both keynotes for these Bowel nosodes.

Follow up: *Four weeks later*
There was still some sensitivity (bloating) to salicylates, but no nasal itching afterwards. Energy levels were better. Constipation was improving.

Prescription 4
Amoxicillin 30: One dose per day for five days. Then continue *Nux vom 30* and *Stannum met* 200 as above. The former was chosen as another intercurrent, because of the frequent use of antibiotics in the patient's history. I considered that 'never well since antibiotics' was an obstacle to cure.

Follow up: *Four weeks later*
Constipation was improved, with passing stool easily every second day. Generally her depressive moods were better. No diarrhoea or bloating.

Prescription 5
Bryonia 200: One dose every second day. (A constipation-specific medicine is now tried.) Introduce some salicylates to assess current level of sensitivity.

Follow up: *Six weeks later*
Initially there was a return of the diarrhoea symptoms (twice shortly after discontinuing the *Nux vom* and *Stannum met)* but the constipation improved, with complete bowel motions most days. *The tolerance to salicylates was improved, with no symptoms on a challenge test.*

Continue *Bryonia 200:* One dose every third day.

Follow up: *Six weeks later*
Apart from one episode of bloating and abdominal pain, and two bouts of diarrhoea (liquid stools), the patient was well. She described herself as "driven ...never satisfied... always looking ahead...had to be the first in class when at school"

Itchy throat still occurs occasionally.
No hayfever symptoms, even after patting cats which normally brings on hayfever).
[*Arsenicum* is noted as a possible constitutional, given the patient's comments about her competitive nature.]

Continue *Bryonia 200:* One dose every fourth day.

Follow up: *Eight weeks later*
All abdominal symptoms have gone. The patient is feeling well except she now has *a return of old symptoms*: gastric reflux. This had been corrected by lapband surgery a few years earlier, with cyclic, episodic reflux still occurring on occasions. She now has noticed a complete return of gastric symptoms.

She described her reflux as dry gagging and retching, worse at night, aggravated by banana and other fruit, temporarily relieved by burping or drinking water. The pain was retro-sternal, radiating to her sides or back. *This was the return of an old symptom.* She had been using *Zantac* since last visit.

The disappearance of presenting symptoms and return of an old symptom is a welcome sign. Now a new prescription is needed to meet the current symptom picture. I choose *Arsenicum* because (i) it matches her constitutional picture and (ii) there is a history of peptic and duodenal ulcer. Since there is a history of peptic ulcer, *Anacardium* is added (see p 76).

Prescription 6
Arsenicum 3: Two doses on one day, alternating with: *Anacardium 200:* One dose on the alternate day.

Follow up: *Six weeks later*
Gastric symptoms completely cleared. No abdominal symptoms returned at all. The only remaining symptom, which had never completely cleared, was the rectal and post nasal itching. Accordingly the last prescription is given to cover these symptoms only.

Prescription 7
Teucrium 200: One dose every second day.

Follow up: Six weeks later

The patient is symptom free. She feels well, with no gastric or abdominal symptoms, and her moods are better. Now she asks me about whether homeopathy may be useful for treating anxiety and depression. In my discussions about what homeopathy can and cannot do, I recommend that she commence psychotherapy simultaneously with my treatment.

Prescription 8

Then I begin treating her with *Arsenicum 200* at two doses per week. I have a number of medicines in mind for her, as the case continues to open up, including *Aurum* and possibly *Diamond Immersion.*

From the perspective her IBS treatment, Felicity is now symptom-free. I would always treat a patient in this sequence: namely (i) treat gut pathology first to 'peel off' that disease layer. Then (ii) move into deeper emotional pathology once that becomes differentiated from physical pathology, and of course, only if requested by the patient.

Discussion

- IBS patients presenting with a history of gastroenteritis are those most likely to have intestinal parasites. This factor, combined with her itching nose and rectal itch, were confirming symptoms. The *Lycopodium* was added because of her symptom severity and the desire to give the patient immediate relief from the bloating. *Cina* and *Lycopodium* are complementary medicines.

- The patient progressed well through giving a number of medicines:
- *Nux vom* and *Stannum met* were chosen because of the ongoing abdominal pain and incomplete evacuation.

- *Bryonia* was chosen when constipation became the remaining dominant symptom. This medicine is discussed at p 79 for the treatment of chronic constipation.

- *Morgan Bowel nosodes* were given to advance the case, based on the patient's depressive moods and abdominal congestion.

- *Amoxicillin* was given as an intercurrent based on the patient's long history of antibiotic use, to remove any possible 'Never well since' obstacle to cure.

- *Arsenicum* and *Anacardium,* are the primary medicines used for peptic ulcer and these were given when those symptoms returned. *Arsenicum* was also considered to be a good choice for her constitution. The return of pre-surgery symptoms after the removal of her current symptoms is consistent with the correct direction of cure, in Hering's Law.

- *Teucrium* was used to conclude the case, given the residual particular post-nasal and rectal symptoms.

- My observation is that long-term abdominal pain, especially if associated with parasitosis, produces profound emotional disturbance.

- I always prescribe on the exact presenting symptoms because they are what the vital force shows us that it needs. Treating in this way is rewarding since the patient feels that their symptoms are getting better at each visit. If they do not feel this, they are likely to lose confidence in the treatment and move on to yet another practitioner. As Felicity's year of treatment progressed, she consistently felt more positive about herself as she experienced her symptoms getting 'lighter'. This is a good indication of the direction of cure taking place. I would only change this prescribing approach if the patient is not feeling better in themselves with treatment.

Case 13: Parasitosis, Sinusitis & Chronic Anxiety

Jane, Female, 29, presented with these symptoms:
Fatigue; abdominal bloating; anxiety; constipation and diarrhoea.
Chronic sinus symptoms with nasal blockage., better first thing in the morning, then gets worse during the day.
Hungry all the time.
Worse after eating.
Rectal and occasionally nasal itch.
My impression is that she is a very anxious patient. She lies awake planning the next day's details. If there is a slight unexpected event in the day it throws her into severe anxiety. I think it unlikely that parasitosis is causing her lifelong anxiety, but I decide to peel off that layer first, so that her constitutional medicine will be clear.

History

Lower back injury with multiple medical procedures.
Panic attacks following back injury.
Eczema.
Childhood insomnia.

Mentals & Generals

Fear in water, in a crowd.
Very anxious when attending social gatherings.
Fear is felt in the epigastrium, "as if I've done something wrong".
Insomnia.

Family History

Mother: hypertension.
Father: hypertension; psoriasis.
Grandmother: cervical cancer.
Grandfather: diabetes, stomach cancer.

Medications

Dithiazide (diuretic)

Prescription 1

Teucrium 200 and *Lycopodium 30:* One dose of each on alternate days. *Gentian & Chelidonium tincture*: 15 drops twice daily. Restrict gluten in diet.

I chose *Teucrium* because she has strong sinus symptoms and I want to remove any possible parasitic cause of symptoms. I also use *Lycopodium* to relieve her abdominal bloating.

Follow up: Four weeks later
There was an improvement in all the symptoms: bloating, sleep, sinus, hunger and anxiety,

Continue *Teucrium 200*: One dose every second day. Use *Lycopodium 30* as needed. Continue *Gentian & Chelidonium tincture*, 15 drops twice daily.

Follow up: Six weeks later
The patient's energy levels and anxiety improved. Her sleep was disturbed, perhaps as a result of still having small amounts of gluten in the diet. She had some sinus: sore throat, puffy sinuses, a minor frontal headache. She was straining at stool followed by some flatulence.

Prescription 2
Dysentery Co 200, single dose; followed by *Trichinose Nosode 30*: one dose every second day. Continue *Gentian & Chelidonium tincture*: 15 drops twice daily. I chose the Bowel nosode *Gaertner* because it is indicated for anticipatory anxiety with gut disturbance.

Follow up: Six weeks later
After the single dose of *Dysentery Co 200*, the blocked nose was initially clear, then blocked on one side only. The bloating and the diarrhoea improved, and the patient could tolerate small amounts of gluten in the diet. The anxiety and poor sleep were still troubling.

Prescription 3
Carcinosin 30: One dose every second day. Her tremendous anxiety where she cannot rest if things are not in order, her childhood (and current) insomnia and family history of cancer suggest this medicine.

Follow up: Four weeks later
Carcinosin had improved her sleep by 80 per cent. She fell asleep easily and if waking, returned to sleep with ease. In the previous visit

I had asked about her childhood. Since then she has thought more about it and describes this story:
In Year Four her schoolteacher was a 'dragon', who frequently made her stand up in front of the class and proceeded to berate her. She felt anxious and embarrassed when recalling the events. Consequently she does not like to be the centre of attention. She feels too embarrassed and self conscious to speak before a group of people. She even had to decline a request to read a poem at the funeral of a close loved one.

Prescription 4
Staphysagria 200: One dose every second day for two weeks.

Follow up: four weeks later
The patient reported a further improvement in her anxiety. She attended two social functions without the usual panic and gut symptoms. Her sinus and diarrhoea had resolved. However, her sleep was still disturbed.

Describing her anxiety, Jane says 'Anything I haven't done before. I don't have the confidence for anything new. I've got to have a structure and plan my day carefully. I'm so shy when in company and feel sure I'll say something stupid'. She is terrified of public speaking. The anxiety she describes is fear of anticipated ordeals and lack of confidence. This suggests *Silicea* which, combined with her history of diarrhoea and the reaction to gluten, suggest the medicine *Gaertner,* which is noted as a future treatment option. However, considering her great response from *Carcinosin,* I decide to continue that treatment in a higher potency.

Prescription 5
Carcinosin 200: One dose every second day for one month.

Follow up: Four weeks later
Her sleep and anxiety are 'fantastic'. Her sleep and bowel symptoms are still triggered by too much gluten, but she can now tolerate small amounts. My treatment plan is to keep her on *Carcinosin* in slowly ascending potencies, while keeping gluten out of her diet for some months. Since her reactivity to gluten is improving, it is likely that it will completely resolve in time if it is excluded.

Discussion

- This patient's gluten sensitivity greatly improved on homeopathic treatment.

- Both *Teucrium* and *Trichinose nosode* were prescribed on a suspected parasitic aetiology. The rectal and nasal itch suggested *Teucrium. Lycopodium* was initially added to offer the patient immediate relief of the discomfort caused by the bloating.

- *Dysentery Co* was chosen as an intercurrent medicine. It was selected because of her history of anticipatory anxiety.

- This is a case where we see the mental symptoms having a direct relationship with the IBS symptoms. The anxiety and insomnia were greatly improved on *Carcinosin* (history of insomnia in children) but the history of embarrassment at school and its consequent effect on her adult self also was helped by *Staphysagria,* which also improved the IBS symptoms. However, she still suffered from loose stools if she ingested too much gluten.

- Would the IBS symptoms have improved if *Staphysagria* been given at the start of the case? I do not think so, since it is not a medicine which shows any antiparasitic action in its *Materia Medica*. But it certainly improved the patient's state of anxiety and embarrassment.

- The patient was asked to undergo a gliadin antibody test to rule out coeliac, despite major improvement in her sensitivity to it.

Chapter 5
Choosing the Order of Treatment

This concise summary of the IBS categories is placed with the recommended treatment priority.

Treatment Priority

Where does one start treatment? For example, a patient may have symptoms suggestive of intestinal parasites (Category 1) but also have an inappropriate diet (Category 12) and anxiety (Category 3).

1. Where there are evident symptoms, or a pathology report, confirming the presence of intestinal parasites, I suggest commencing treatment with eradication of the parasites. In the above example, one would thus give a medicine such as *Cina* plus some advice about diet and lifestyle. If the anxiety requires further treatment, then once the symptoms caused by the parasite are cleared, the need for a medicine for anxiety alone will become evident, and that medicine can be given later.

2. The second treatment priority is a 'never well since' causation, for example never well since Infectious Mononucleosis. Prescribe an antidote to that causation (eg *Coxsackievirus, Glandular Fever Nosode, Carcinosin* or other specific homeopathic medicine*) before* giving the constitutional medicine. In my experience, a constitutional medicine will not be effective if there is an exogenous disease phenomenon, which will block the action of the constitutional medicine.

3. Next, I suggest a medicine which is specific for the presenting symptoms, focusing carefully on the particulars, and how those particulars are influenced by the general characteristics of the patient. To determine which symptoms to focus on, I usually ask the patient what is worrying them the most right now. Their answer will in most cases focus me to what needs treatment next. For example, 'my constipation gives me pain in the right upper tummy, and is always worse when I become overheated'.

4. When the *particular* symptoms that are *influenced by the generals* are better, it is time to focus on a constitutional or 'mentals' treatment, *if that is what the patient wants.*

5. If the patient fails to recover fully after the above treatment priority there may be a crucial symptom from the history which has been missed, or perhaps there is a pathology which requires investigation. Alternatively, the idea of 'cellular memory', as described in Category 15, may be relevant.

I have found it most effective to prescribe on the exact presenting symptoms because they are what the vital force shows us that it needs. Treating in this way is rewarding since the patient feels that their symptoms are getting better at each visit. If they do not feel this, they are likely to lose confidence in the treatment and move on to yet another practitioner. Provided the patient feels better within themselves, this is a good indication of the direction of cure taking place. I would only change this prescribing approach if the patient is not feeling better in himself with treatment.

A useful example of the method of treatment priority is illustrated by Case 12 at p 126. Treatment priority is therefore (by way of example):

1. Intestinal Parasites......*Cina*
2. 'Never well since'......*Coxsackievirus*
3. Specific presenting symptoms, eg a specific medicine for constipation.
4. Mentals or generals prescription, eg a medicine for anxiety.
5. Cellular memory or another factor.

Where a patient does not appear to fit into any of these categories, or the medicines selected fail to achieve improvement in symptoms, next consider one of the Bowel nosodes, or one of the medicines for symptom particulars. If these measures fail, re-take the case!

Categories and Treatment Priority

Category 1: Intestinal Parasitosis
Treatment Priority: 1
Pain, constipation, diarrhoea, food sensitivity, rectal itch, emotional disturbance associated with symptoms

Category 2: Candida
Treatment Priority: 3
History of vaginal or oral thrush, intestinal bloating, sugar aggravation, history of antibiotic use

Category 3: Emotional Disturbance
Treatment Priority: 4
Anxiety, anger, depression, especially if withheld, will all affect the gastro-intestinal system.

Category 4: Food Sensitivity
Treatment Priority: 3
Aggravation from certain foods only: most commonly wheat, gluten, dairy, salicylate. Investigate possible coeliac disease.

Category 5: 'Never well since'
Treatment Priority: 2
Clear aetiology requires specific antidote.

Category 6: Gastric Reflux
Treatment Priority: 3
Heartburn, regurgitation, scratchy throat or aphonia.

Category 7: Gallbladder Stasis
Treatment Priority: 3
Nausea and inability to digest fatty food, with possible pale stool.

Category 8: Gastritis &/or Peptic Ulcer
Treatment Priority: 3
Epigastric pain after meals, sometimes with acid belching.

Category 9: Post-viral
Treatment Priority: 2
Fatigue, recurring colds and influenzas, sleep disturbance, fevers.

Category 10: Constipation
Treatment Priority: 3
Constipation with or without abdominal pain.

Category 11: Diarrhoea
Treatment Priority: 3
Simple diarrhoea, while more likely caused by intestinal parasites, has a variety of other causes.

Category 12: Diet and Lifestyle Factors:
Treatment Priority: 2
Check nutrition and lifestyle factors.

Category 13: Bowel nosodes
Treatment Priority: 3

Category 14: Particulars only
Treatment Priority: 3

Category 15: CNS Memory
Treatment Priority: 5

Chapter 6
A Parasitic Miasm

Miasm
When a well-selected medicine fails to act, we think of a chronic miasm. Hahnemann originally identified three miasms, while more have been described since his original work *The Chronic Diseases.* A miasm (literally 'infection') means a hidden, chronic, and disease-producing influence which prevents a well-selected medicine being effective, or causes the symptoms to relapse, until such time as an 'anti-miasmatic' medicine is chosen to treat that miasm. There are seven generally accepted miasms, which have recently been researched by Grant Bentley.[29] They are:

- Psora
- Sycosis
- Syphilis
- Syco-Psora
- Syco-Syphilis
- Tuberculosis
- Cancer

Many more miasmatic suggestions have been made by Rajan Sankaran[30] and others as the knowledge of microbiology expands.

Parasitic Miasm
If a miasm is a hidden, chronic, disease-producing influence, then the wide range of symptoms described for intestinal parasitosis represents a miasm. Many medicines afford symptomatic relief of parasite-generated symptoms, but those will not rid the body of parasites until a specific anti-parasitic medicine is used, which is prescribed on the presenting symptoms. In clinic I have found that the four medicines described Chapter 3 for the treatment of a parasitic miasm are, in almost all cases, all that are needed to start improvement in even the most obstinate cases.

---

[29] Bentley, G, Appearance and Circumstance: Miasms, Facial Features and Homeopathy, Pennon Publishing, Melbourne, 2003

[30] See, for example, *The Substance of Homeopathy,*4th ed, Homeopathic Medical Publishers, Mumbai, 1999.

While this is a surprisingly short list of medicines, it is in keeping with Hahnemann's findings on the treatment of the Chronic Miasms. Hahnemann used *Sulphur*, sometimes *Psorinum*, to treat the Psoric Miasm: essentially just two medicines! Many patients with IBS do not improve significantly without an anti-parastic medicine.

Patients with digestive disease often do not respond to a well-chosen medicine. Example: you prescribe *Argentum nit* for anticipatory diarrhoea, but it does not help. You may deduce that it is the patient's anxiety which is producing the diarrhoea. But if one considers the effect of anxiety on the vital force, whatever disease one has (whether, for example, migraines, heartburn or diarrhoea) anxiety will always turn up the volume on those symptoms. Anxiety is a modifying factor, or a trigger of a latent condition, *but it may not be the cause*. In such a case, *Argentum nit* will not work since anxiety is not the chief cause of the diarrhoea, *but an aggravating factor*. The cause may be intestinal parasites. *Cina* treats diarrhoea with anxiety where there is intestinal parasitosis. *In my experience, a constitutional medicine will not work if a physical pathology is present. One must first use a specific treatment for that physical pathology of intestinal parasitosis, which I identify as a chronic miasm.* If by coincidence the constitutional medicine is also an anti-parasitic, then two disease phenomena (constitution and parasitosis) can be addressed with that medicine, but this is a rare occurrence.

Unusual symptoms caused by intestinal parasitosis
Many symptoms other than gastrointestinal ones can be caused by the parasitic miasm. One would not necessarily think of intestinal parasitosis when one sees:

- Emotional disturbance: irritability and/or anxiety
- Rectal, nasal or palate itching
- Sinus symptoms or "allergies"
- Teeth grinding (patients attribute this to their anxiety)
- Disturbed sleep, including night terrors in children, insomnia in adults
- Chronic post nasal symptoms with thick, purulent mucus
- Headaches.

My current thinking on the parasitic miasm explains why IBS patients with some of the above symptoms do not respond to a well-selected homeopathic medicine. It also explains why the action of the well-chosen medicine does not endure. How many insomnia patients with some gastro-intestinal disturbance might need *Cina*? It is easy as a homeopath to focus on insomnia or irritability as having an entirely emotional cause. There are many examples of exogenous phenomena, like pathogens, affecting emotions. As homeopaths, we are well accustomed to pathogens causing a plethora of mental and emotional symptoms; even simple scabies (a skin parasite) can produce depression and anxiety: take a look at *Psorinum*!

Gastric Reflux

One may well question how so many different gastro-intestinal symptoms can be caused by intestinal parasitosis. Gastro-oesophageal reflux, for example, sometimes occurs in IBS patients. I have found that giving an anti-parasitic medicine sometimes improves the reflux. What does this mean? How do intestinal parasites cause reflux? Earlier homeopaths, such as Dr Charles Fisher,[31] suggest that parasites can survive in the gastric juices of the stomach and cause dyspepsia. One of the more unusual cases presented in this book, Case 3, suggests this may be possible.

It may also be possible that chronic inflammation, muscle spasm or other functional damage to the gut wall, from whatever cause, may leave lasting effects on the nervous tissue. This may be caused by toxins produced by the gut pathogens and may cause the inappropriate opening of cardiac sphincter. In other words, reflux may be the result of:

- Actual presence of parasites in the gastric acid (according to Fisher), or
- Toxins produced by the gut parasites affect the nervous system.

I have seen in clinic that local (eg abdominal spasm) and regional (eg headaches) disturbances in the nervous system respond well to treatment for parasitosis. The effect of parasitosis may well include many other symptoms of functional disturbance which have not yet been identified. The greater the involvement of the nervous system

[31] Fisher, CE, *A Hand-book on the Diseases of Children and Their Homeopathic Treatment*(1895), B Jain Publishers, New Delhi, 1997

(ie nervous or emotional symptoms) in parasitosis, the more appropriate it is to prescribe *Cina* as the first medicine.

Parasite transmission to humans

There is a myriad of ways that parasite eggs and cysts are transmitted to humans:

- No or inadequate hand washing before eating or touching the mouth
- Inadequate hygiene around domestic pets
- Eating undercooked meat
- Sharing your meal with a child (who has had contact with other children harboring parasites)
- Kissing
- Contaminated water supply (cryptosporidium was detected in the Sydney water catchment in 1999)
- Walking barefoot especially in tropical climates (eg dog hookworm)
- Eating unwashed, unpeeled fruit (touched by someone else who has cysts on their fingers)
- Normal hand to mouth contact[32].

More serious effects of parasites

There can be more serious consequences if parasites migrate from the intestinal tract to the liver or brain. For example, Taenia oncospheres can migrate to the brain (causing epilepsy). Toxoplasmosis, if acquired during pregnancy, can migrate through the placenta and affect the child's eyes (chorioretinitis) and brain (convulsions, hydrocephaly, psychomotor disturbances). These cases are comparatively fortunately rare.

Who is likely to have intestinal parasites?

As homeopaths we speak generally about individual susceptibility, but there is a more specific way in which one develops susceptibility to gut parasites: gut dysbiosis. Dysbiosis is the disturbance to the normal beneficial bowel flora which permits the growth of pathogenic bacteria, viruses, fungi and parasites. It is widely acknowledged that dysbiosis is caused by:

---

[32] See the Center for Disease Control factsheets and guidelines: www.cdc.gov/ncdod/dpd/parasitesamebiasis/fctsht

- Overuse of antibiotics
- The oral contraceptive pill
- Long term use of corticosteroids
- Diets which have excess amounts of carbohydrates, sugars, food colourings and preservatives
- Long term stress.

Healing the Dysbiotic Gut

In gut environments where there is chronic inflammation and/or leaky gut syndrome (ie an increase in permeability of the intestinal mucosa to luminal macromolecules, antigens and toxins associated with inflammatory degenerative and/or atrophic mucosal damage [33]), removal of the food triggers is essential.

The food triggers often involve:

- Gluten, and in severe cases all grains
- Starchy vegetables (which prevent healing of the gut in some cases)
- Unfermented milk products (eg ordinary milk)
- Eggs
- Salicylates
- Any food to which the patient is sensitive!

Dietary factors & obstacle to cure

When dietary error is a factor it must be considered to be an obstacle to cure. The patient will need foods high in essential fatty acids such as meat, fish, poultry, eggs, butter. Fermented foods which contain lactobacilli are helpful in correcting the dysbiosis: this includes natural yoghurt, sauerkraut, pickles and kefir.[34] At the time of writing we are trialling kefir hand-succussed to a 3X potency to attempt to stimulate lactobacilli production in patients with chronic dysbiosis.

A prolonged diet of refined carbohydrates, take away and convenience meals with food additives and preservatives, and foods lacking essential vitamins and minerals, adversely impact on health. These dietary factors must be considered as obstacles to

[33] See for example, Campbell-McBride, N, *Gut and Psychology Syndrome,* Medinform Publishing, Cambridge, UK, 2004

[34] Ibid

homeopathic cure. The best selected medicine cannot correct dietary deficiencies.

Some common examples of nutritional deficiency are:

- B12 deficiency in vegetarians (especially vegans)
- Iron deficiency in menstruating women and vegetarian
- Poor mineral absorption in patients who have either hypochlorhydria or gut dysbiosis
- B-group vitamins do not synthesise in gut dysbiosis so many patients need B-group supplementation.

How to determine Parasitosis

- On symptoms alone
- Digestive stool test, as described in Chapter 1.
- Applied kinesiology (muscle testing against pathogen samples)
- Electro-dermal testing.

Of these tests, only a digestive stool analysis performed by skilled pathologists will give a definitive diagnosis. However, when one has seen many cases of intestinal parasitosis, it becomes more easily identifiable on symptoms alone.

Chapter 7
Frequently Asked Questions

Q. Does everyone who has intestinal parasites have IBS?

A. No. There are individual factors such as heredity, predisposition, constitution, environment, etc. Some individuals who have intestinal parasites are asymptomatic.

Q. Does everyone with IBS have intestinal parasites?

A. No. Approximately 70 per cent of IBS patients have intestinal parasites.

Q. Does the one particular parasitic organism cause the same type of IBS symptoms in every individual?

A. No, every person responds to a parasite in a different way, and thus has different symptoms. However, those symptoms can generally be grouped into one of the *Materia Medica* of one the treatment protocols described for intestinal parasitosis.

Q. If you have a case where you identify a constitutional medicine, along with a 'never well since', plus you determine the presence of intestinal parasites, which treatment should you give first?

A. 1. Eradicate the intestinal parasites. 2. Address the 'never well since'. 3. The constitutional medicine.

Q. Why are the recommended homeopathic medicines repeated so often and in some cases for many months?

A. Dr John Paterson said, "The clearing of threadworms is difficult and usually requires prolonged treatment".[35] This concurs with my

[35] Paterson, J, *The Bowel Nosodes,* B Jain Publishers, New Delhi, 1988, p 6; reprinted from *The British Homeopathic Journal*, Vol XL, No 3, July 1950

clinical experience where symptoms easily relapse without prolonged treatment. I use an anti-parasitic medicine every second day for at least one month and in some cases many months. This frequent repetition not only expels the parasite, but alters the dynamic sensitivity of the patient to parasitosis and reduces the likelihood of re-infestation.

Q. Will a constitutional medicine get rid of parasites?

A. No. The parasites are *exogenous pathogens which form a chronic miasm, resulting in an impediment to cure*. There are only a small number of known homeopathic medicines which have an anti-parasitic action. The individual symptoms still show us which medicines to use. An anti-parasitic medicine should be given before constitutional treatment.

Dr Charles Fisher's experience of treating children with worms further explains what I have described here.[36]

Q. When choosing the medicine, does it matter what kind of intestinal parasite the patient has?

A. No. Choose the medicine based on the presenting symptoms, irrespective of the type of parasite.

Q. Can one use intestinal parasite medicines such as Cina for the treatment of acute traveler's diarrhoea or gastroenteritis?

A. No. Acute medicines are required for acute conditions. The treatment protocols for intestinal parasitosis described in Chapter 3 are for chronic disease. Acute medicines such as *Arsenicum, Aloe, Mercurius cor, Veratrum alb, Lycopodium, Podophyllum* etc should be used for acute treatment.

Q. Can one use lactobacilli supplements to correct gut dysbiosis and thereby eradicate intestinal parasites?

---

[36] Fisher, CE, *A Hand-book on the Diseases of Children and Their Homeopathic Treatment*(1895), B Jain Publishers, New Delhi, 1997, p 559.

A. No. Lactobacilli supplements will only be of value once the parasites have been eradicated, and restoration of normal gut flora is then desired. Lactobacilli supplements may maintain beneficial flora, but they are not an anti-parasitic treatment. Bowel treatment with probiotics requires therapeutic doses of a range of organisms for prolonged periods.

Q. Why can't one treat a patient's anxiety with a specific medicine for their anxiety before commencing an anti-parasitic treatment?

A. You can, but the affect may be short-lived or ineffective. The gut or parasitic symptoms need to be differentiated from the emotional disturbance. This process can change the presentation of the emotional disturbance, revealing a more accurate medicine. Good case-taking and an accurate analysis of the symptoms are essential. Are the mental or emotional symptoms accompanied by gut symptoms? What is the origin of the anxiety?

Appendix 1

Rome II Diagnostic Criteria for IBS:

At least 12 weeks (which need not be consecutive) in the preceding 12 months of abdominal discomfort or pain with two of the following features:

- The abdominal discomfort or pain is relieved with defecation and/or
- the onset is associated with a change in frequency of stools and/or
- the onset associated with a change in the form (appearance) of stool .

Symptoms that cumulatively support the diagnosis of IBS:

- Abnormal stool frequency (perhaps more than 3 bowel movements per day or less than 3 bowel movements per week)
- Abnormal stool form (lumpy/hard or loose/watery)
- Abnormal stool passage (straining, urgency, feeling of incomplete evacuation)
- Passage of mucus
- Bloating or feeling of abdominal distension.

Appendix 2

Common Intestinal Parasites and their Symptoms

Pathogen	Variety	Transmission	Symptoms
Blastocystis hominis	Protozoa	Oral-faecal	• Diarrhoea • Abdominal cramps • Nausea • Vomiting • Abdominal pain • Perianal pruritis • Iron deficiency • Oesinophilia
Dientamoeba fragilis	Flagellate	Oral-faecal	• Diarrhoea • Fatigue • Anorexia • Poor weight gain • Nausea • Abdominal pain • Bloating • Vomiting
Entamoeba histolytica	Flagellate protozoa	Oral-faecal	• Abdominal pain • Diarrhoea • Blood in stools • Chronic colitis
Giardia Lamblia	Protozoa	Oral-faecal	• Diarrhoea • Nausea • Epigastric pain • Weight loss • Malabsorption • Malaise
Cryptosporidium parvum	Protozoa	Oral-faecal	• Diarrhoea • Abdominal pain • Dehydration • Weight loss • Fever • Nausea • Vomiting
Toxoplasmosis gondii	Protozoa	Oral-faecal (under-cooked meat)	• Diarrhoea • Fatigue • Malaise • Lymphadenopathy • Mimics infectious mononucleosis
Balantidium coli	Protozoa	Oral-faecal	• Diarrhoea
Fasciolopsis buski	Fluke	Oral-faecal	• Diarrhoea • Oedema • Abdominal pain
Paragonimus westermani (lung fluke)	Fluke	Oral-faecal – esp crabs & crayfish	• Diarrhoea • Rarely pulmonary symptoms
Brachylaima cribbi	Fluke	Oral-faecal (from snails)	• Diarrhoea
Trichinella spiralis (trichinosis)	Worm	Oral-faecal (under-cooked meat)	• Diarrhoea • Bloating • Rectal itch

Selected Bibliography

Articles

- Haresh, K, et al, *Trop Med Int Health,* 1999; 4:274
- Heap, Timothy, "How to Treat: Irritable Bowel Syndrome", *Australian Doctor,* 23.10.98 & 30.10.98
- Hewett, Peter, "How to Treat: Acute Lower Abdominal Pain", *Australian Doctor,* 14.2.03, I-VIII
- Holten, K, et al, "Diagnosing the patient with abdominal pain and altered bowel habits: is it irritable bowel syndrome?" *Am Fam Physician,* 2003; 67: 2157-62
- Holten, K, et al, "Irritable Bowel Syndrome: minimize testing, let symptoms guide treatment", *J Fam Pract,* 2003; 52: 942-50
- Howlett, M & Gibson, P, "Update: Crohn's Disease", *Medical Observer,* 12.12.03, 28-29.
- Jones, J, et al, "British Society of Gastroenterology guidelines for the management of irritable bowel syndrome", *Gut,* 2000; 47 (supp II): ii-19
- Kennedy, T, et al, "Cognitive Behavioural Therapy in addition to antispasmodic treatment for irritable bowel syndrome in primary care: randomized clinical trial", *British Medical Journal* 2005; 331:435
- Ratnaike, Ranjit, "How to Treat: Constipation", *Australian Doctor,* 17.9.99, I-VIII
- Rieger, Nicholas, "How to Treat: Faecal Incontinence", *Australian Doctor,* 6.9.02, I-VII
- Starr, J, "Clostridium difficile associated diarrhoea: diagnosis and treatment", *British Medical Journal* 2005; 331: 498-501

Books

- Banerji, P & Mukherjee, S, "Little Worms and Little Children with Great Troubles", in *A Few Papers on Clinical Research of Parimal Banerji on Advanced Homeopathic Therapeutics,* Vol 2, Advanced Thinkers, Calcutta, 1996
- Banerji, P, *Advanced Homeopathy & Its Materia Medica,* Advanced Thinkers, Calcutta, 1986
- Berkow, et al, *The Merck Manual, 17th ed,* Merck & Co, NJ,
- Boericke, W, *Pocket Manual of Homeopathic Materia Medica,*9th ed, 1927, B Jain, New Delhi
- Brown, H, *Basic Clinical Parasitology,* Appleton-Century-Crofts, 1975.
- Campbell-Mcbride, N, *Gut and Psychology Syndrome,* Medinform Publishing, Cambridge, UK, 2004
- Clarke, J, *Dictionary of Practical Materia Medica,* London, (1900), B Jain, New Delhi
- Fisher, CE, *A Hand-book on the Diseases of Children and Their Homeopathic Treatment*(1895), B Jain Publishers, New Delhi, 1997

- Gamble, J, *Mastering Homeopathy: Accurate Daily Prescribing for a Successful Practice,* Karuna Publishing, Wollongong, Australia, 2004
- Garcia, L, *Diagnostic Medical Parasitology,* 4th ed, ASM Press, 2001.
- Hahnemann, S., *The Chronic Diseases,* (ed Tafel, Hughes, Dudley), 1896.
- Julian, O, *Treatise on Dynamised Micro Immunotherapy (1977)*, B Jain, New Delhi
- Morrison, R, *Desktop Guide to Keynotes and Confirmatory Symptoms,* Hahnemann Clinic Publishing, CA, 1993
- Paterson, J, *The Bowel Nosodes,* B Jain Publishers, New Delhi, 1988, reprinted from *The British Homeopathic Journal*, Vol XL, No 3, July 1950
- Satsangi, J & Sutherland, L (eds), *Inflammatory Bowel Disease,* Churchill Livingston, London, 2003.
- Sheorey, H et al, *Clinical Parasitology, A Handbook for Medical Practitioners and Microbiologists,* MUP, Melbourne, 2000.
- Smits, Tinus, *Inspiring Homeopathy: the Treatment of Universal Layers,* 1999
- *The Substance of Homeopathy,*4th ed, Homeopathic Medical Publishers, Mumbai, 1999
- Vermuelen, F, *Synoptic Materia Medica, Vols 1 & 2,* Merlijn Publishers, The Netherlands, 6th & 2nd eds (2000 & 1998)

Websites

- www.ksu.edu/parasitology/625tutorials/index.html
- http://www.geocities.com/parasiteatlas/parasites.html
- http://www.cdd.com.au/html/expertise/diseaseinfo/ibs.html

Index of Medicines

Abies nig, 75
Allium-c, 70, 88
Aloe, 80, 86, 98, 148
Alumina, 79
Amoxicillin, 69, 128, 130
Anacardium, 76, 129, 131
Argentum nit, 64, 66, 84, 142
Arsenicum, 65-66, 75, 76, 129, 129-131, 148
Artemesia vulg, 59
Asafoetida, 63, 66, 75, 89
Aurum met, 130
Bacillus No 7, 84
Bryonia, 79, 86, 112-113, 128-130
Calcarea carb, 84
Calcarea phos, 65-66
Camphor, 70
Candida albicans, 61
Carbo veg, 66, 70
Carcinosin, 133-135, 136
Carduus mar, 101
Causticum, 65-66
Chamomilla, 64, 66
Chelidonium, 72-74, 76, 107, 118, 132-133
China, 70
Cina, 12, 52-54, 57-58, 60, 63, 66, 77, 93, 95, 97, 98, 101, 107, 115, 118-119, 127, 130, 136, 137, 142, 143, 144, 148
Colocynthis, 64, 66, 81, 86
Coxsackievirus, 69-70, 78, 110-111, 136, 137
Cuprum met, 89
Diamond Immersion, 130
Dysentery Co, 84, 133, 135
Entamoeba hystolica, 109
Folliculinum, 70, 121-122
Gaertner, 54, 58, 69, 83, 88, 134
Gentian, 72, 132-133
Glandular fever Nosode, 70, 136
Hyoscamus, 88
Ignatia, 66, 76, 84, 88
Indigo, 58
Ipecac, 86
Iris vers, 76
Kreosotum, 61
Lycopodium, 61, 64, 66, 76, 84, 86, 93, 94, 114-115, 125, 127, 130, 132-133, 135, 148
Mercurius cor, 80, 86, 93, 94, 109, 110-111, 148
Mercurius sol, 58, 65-66, 118
Morgan Bach/Pure/Gaertner, 84, 88, 97, 98, 109-110, 127, 130
Natrum mur, 65-66
Natrum phos, 75
Natrum sulph, 84
Nux vom, 13, 53-54, 57, 60, 64, 66, 79, 86, 104-5, 110-111, 127-128, 130
Opium, 65-66, 88
Penicillin, 69, 83
Phosphoric ac, 66
Phosphorus, 63, 66, 83
Plumbum, 79, 86
Podophyllum, 80, 148
Proteus, 84, 88
Psorinum, 142-143
Robinia, 75
Saccharum, 124-125
Silicea, 102-3, 134
Spigelia, 58, 88
Stannum met, 52-54 57, 60, 77, 104-5, 110-111, 127-128, 130
Staphysagria, 70, 88, 115-116, 134-135
Stramonium, 55, 65-66
Sulphur, 58, 142
Sycotic co, 84, 93
Teucrium, 52, 54, 57, 60, 77, 120-121, 129, 131, 132-133, 135
Thuja, 58
Trichinose Nosode, 52, 55, 58, 60, 93, 95, 114-115, 121, 133, 135
Veratrum album, 148
Wheat, 67

General Index

Abdominal pain, 22, 51, 53-55, 57-58, 60-61, 64, 74, 76-77, 80-81, 86-88
Addison's disease, 40
Aerophagy, 40
Aggravation, 56
Allergy, 17, 22, 51, 53-54, 60, 83, 120, 132, 133, 134, 135
Allopathic drugs, 33, 70, 112-113
Anaemia, 17, 22, 41, 45, 47, 51, 54, 60
Anger, 66
Anorexia, 22, 43, 51, 60, 82
Antibiotics, 23, 25, 27, 69, 71, 83
Antidepressants, 18
Anxiety, 12, 18, 22, 24, 25, 47, 51-53, 55, 57, 60, 63-66, 75-76, 79, 84-85, 88-89, 92-95, 114-116, 130, 132, 133, 134, 135
Aphthous ulcer, 42
Appendicitis,40, 48
Appetite, 22, 47, 52, 54
Behavioural problems, children, in, 123-125
Belching, 28, 66, 89
Bloating – see Flatulence
Blood, stool, in, 19, 42, 46-47, 81, 86
Bowel nosodes, 83-85
Brain tumour, 32
Breath offensive, 88
Buccal mucosa irritation, 58
Calculi, 73
Candida albicans, 23, 40-41, 61, 67
Carcinoid syndrome, 41
Carcinoma,
  colonic, 42
  pancreatic, 46
Catarrh, 84
Cauda equine, 32
Cellular memory, 37, 87, 137
Cerebro-vascular accident, 32
Chronic fatigue syndrome, 70, 78, 84, 110, 111
Cholecystitis, 100, 101
Clinkers, 54
Coeliac disease, 41, 52, 58, 67, 105
Cognitive Behavioural Therapy, 24
Colds & flues, 31, 77
Colitis,
  haemorrhagic, 45
  ischaemic, 46, 48
  ulcerative, 47
Colonoscopy, 17, 59
Constipation, 22, 25, 32-33, 41, 43, 51-54, 60, 63, 79-80, 84, 86, 88-89, 112-113, 126, 127
Constitutional treatment, 50, 59, 63, 69
Cough, 30, 75
Crawling sensation, 53, 60
Crohn's disease, 43, 86
Cytomegalo virus 77
Dementia, 32
Depression, 32, 42, 84-85, 88, 126, 128, 130
Diabetes, 33, 65, 88
Diarrhoea, 25, 34, 40-41, 43, 46-48, 51-53, 55, 60, 63-66, 70, 77, 79-81, 83-84, 86, 89, 92-95, 126, 127
Diet, IBS, in, 18, 35
Diverticulitis, 43, 48
Dizziness, 61
Dynamis 50
Dysbiosis, 11, 20-21, 23, 25, 32, 34, 61-62, 83
Dysphagia, 28, 30, 71, 75
Ectopic pregnancy, 44
Eczema, 85
Emaciation, 51, 54, 60, 85
Embolic injury, 43
Epstein-Barr virus, 77-78
Eructation see Belching
Exogenous disease, 50
Faecal incontinence, 80, 86, 123
Fastidious, 88
Fatigue, 17, 23, 31, 41-42, 47, 51, 60, 61, 77-78, 85
Fever, 17, 22, 40, 43, 44-46, 52, 60
Flatulence, 22, 23, 28, 30, 40-41, 51, 60, 61-64, 66, 70, 75-76, 126, 127, 128, 132, 133, 134, 135
Flushes of heat, 22, 51, 53, 60
Food sensitivity or intolerance, 25-26, 29, 67, 72, 80
Gallbladder
  colic 100, 101
  stasis, 29, 67, 72-73, 106, 107
Gastric ulcer see Peptic ulcer
Gastritis, 30, 65, 75-76

Gastroenteritis, 58, 69, 92-95, 117-118
Gastro-oesophageal reflux, 28, 41, 63, 71, 75-76, 82, 88-89, 129
Glandular fever, 27, 65, 69-70, 77-78, 110
Grief, 65, 66
Growing pains, 65
Guilt, 66
Gut flora – see Dysbiosis
Haemorrhoids, 48
Headache, 17, 29, 31, 40, 41, 58, 59, 61, 65, 72, 77, 92-95
Heartburn, 28, 30, 72, 75
Heavy metal toxicity, 79
Helicobacter pylori, 71, 117
Hering's law, 101, 102, 103, 131
Hernia,
    hiatus, 64
    inguinal, 45
Homeopathic medicine ineffective, 57
see also Posology; Obstacle to cure
Hunger, 88
Hypercalcaemia, 33
Hyperchlorhydria, 71
Hypersensitive, 85, 88
Hypochlorhydria, 28, 30, 67, 71-73
Hypoglycaemia, 61, 67
Hypokalaemia, 33
Hypotension, 40
Hysteria, 64, 66, 75, 85, 88, 100
Iatrogenic, 96-98
Impediment to cure, 50
Indifference, 66
Inflammatory bowel disease, 45
Injury, 87
Insomnia, 12, 17, 22, 51, 54, 55, 60, 65, 88, 92-95, 114, 115, 132, 133, 134, 135
Intestinal parasites see Parasites, intestinal
Introspection, 84, 85
Irritability, 22, 52, 55, 57, 60, 64, 85
Itch,
    nasal, 22, 52, 60
    rectal, 22,52-54, 60, 88
    skin, 22, 52, 60
Kefir, 62, 68
Lactobacilli, 11
Laxatives, 79
Leaky gut, 25-26, 83
Leg pain, 58
Leucorrhoea, 61
Lump in throat, 30, 75
Malabsorption, 41-42, 58, 83,
Malignancy, 88
Manning Criteria, 16
Materia medica, 52, 102
Miasm, chronic, 56, Parasitic, 56
    Sycotic, 84
Mittelschmerz, 44
Monilia, see Candida albicans
Mononucleosis see Glandular Fever
Mood swings, 23, 41, 61, 64
Multiple sclerosis
Myalgia, 31, 77
Nasal polyp, 54, 60
Nausea, 17, 22, 29, 31, 52, 59-60, 72, 77-78, 88
'Never well since', 27, 65, 69-70, 108-111, 116, 121, 136
Night terrors, 22, 52, 54-55, 60, 63
Obstacle to cure, 50, 63, 69, 82, 121
Obstruction, bowel, 46, 48
Oral contraceptive pill, 27, 70
Osteoporosis, 42
Ovarian
    Cancer, 44
    cyst, 44
Palpitations, 58, 88
Parasites,
    children and, 22, 104-105
    constipation and, 22
    gastroenteritis, and 20
    herbal medicine in treatment of,59
    intestinal, 20-22,51-60, 63, 87, 92-95, 136
    see also Miasm, Parasitic
Parasitosis, see Parasites
Parkinson's disease, 32
Pathology, treatment of, 55
Peptic ulcer, 30, 65, 73, 76, 131
Peritonitis, 46, 48
Porphyria,33
Posology, 55, 57
Post-nasal drip, 54
Priority of treatment, 136-139
Recreational drugs, 82
'Red flag' symptoms, 17, 19
Reflux, gastric see Gastro-oesophageal reflux
Regurgitation, 28, 30, 63, 71, 84, 89

Rectal prolapse, 34, 46
Restless Leg Syndrome, 17, 22, 52-53, 60
Salivation, 58
Salpingitis, 44
Shy, 85
Shy-Drager Syndrome
Sinusitis see Allergy
Sleep, disturbed, see Night terrors; Insomnia
Sleepwalking, 59, 63
Sluggishness, 53
Spastic colon, 19
Spinal cord lesions, 32
Squint, 58
Stammer, 88
Steatorrhoea, 41, 52
Stool, Diagnostic, test, 20-21
Stool, pale, 72-73
Stress see Anxiety
Sugar cravings, 23, 61
Suppression, 56-57
Surgery, 70, 80, 87, 89
Tachycardia, 47
Tautopathy, 69
Teeth clenching / grinding, 22, 52-53, 55, 60
Tonsillitis or pharyngitis, 77, 88
Throat tightness, 71
Thrush, 23, 41, 61
Thyroid disease, 33, 41, 47
Urinary tract infection, 44
Violence, 65, 85
Viral, post, 31, 77-78, 84, 108-111
Voice loss, 75
Vomiting, 40, 53, 65, 76, 84, 88
Weakness, 22, 52, 60
Weight loss, 17, 22, 42-43, 46-47, 52, 54, 60, 83
Zollinger-Ellison Syndrome, 47

Acknowledgements

I am greatly indebted to my wife and partner, Nyema Hermiston for compiling much of the medical research material used in this work and also for sub-editing the text. My cumbersome grammar was thereby transformed into something far more readable.

Thank you to Helen McGuire for writing up and editing the case studies from my original case notes, and for revising the manuscript on two occasions.

John Maitland and Patricia Janssen were also kind enough to revise the first proof of this book.

Thank you to Peter Tumminello for writing the Foreword.

Dr Parimal Banerji's for his methods of prescribing and his knowledge of *Materia Medica* in which he defines the optimum potencies for some of the medicines I frequently use, have also influenced this work.

To all the Australian homeopaths from whom I have learned pearls of wisdom over the years, I give thanks. Among them are David Levy, Ken D'Aran, Alastair Gray, Peter Tumminello and Alan Jones.